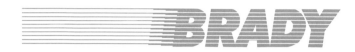

Pediatric Emergencies

A Manual for Prehospital Care Providers

Second Edition

Martin R. Eichelberger, M.D.

Jane W. Ball, R.N., Dr. P.H.

Geraldine L. Pratsch, R.N., M.P.H.

John R. Clark, NREMT-P

BRADY
Prentice Hall
Upper Saddle River, New Jersey 07458

Library of Congress Cataloging-in-Publication Data

Brady pediatric emergencies : a manual for prehospital care providers
/ Martin R. Eichelberger . . . [et al.]. — 2nd ed.
    p.   cm
  Includes bibliographical references and index.
  ISBN 0-8359-5123-5
    1. Pediatric emergencies—Handbooks, manuals, etc. 2. Pediatric
emergency services—Handbooks, manuals, etc.   I. Eichelberger,
Martin.
    [DNLM: 1. Emergencies—in infancy & childhood—handbooks.
2. Accidents—in infancy & childhood—handbooks. WS 39 P3706 1997]
RJ370.P4264 1997
618.92′ 0025—dc21
DNLM/DLC
for Library of Congress   97-6025
                                                                  CIP

Publisher: Susan Katz
Director of production/manufacturing: Bruce Johnson
Managing production editor: Patrick Walsh
Editorial/production supervision: Janet McGillicuddy
Project editor/interior design: Barbara J. Barg, Navta
    Associates, Inc.
Electronic art specialist: Robin Lucas
Cover design: Bruce Kenselaar
Cover photo: PhotoDisc, Inc.
Prepress/manufacturing buyer: Ilene Sanford
Editorial sssistant: Carol Sobel

This text is dedicated to all Prehospital Providers and the children and families in their care.

Prehospital Providers continue to be champions in changing the EMS system to accommodate the child. We salute all of you in your professionalism and dedication!

This book was previously published
under the title *Pediatric Emergencies Manual*,
M.R. Eichelberger and G. Stossel-Pratsch, eds.,
Rockville, MD: Aspen Publishers, 1984.

Chapter 4 was contributed by
Michael McAdams, NREMT-P.

Printed in the United States of America
10 9 8 7 6 5 4 3 2 1

ISBN 0-8359-5123-5

Prentice-Hall International (UK) Limited, *London*
Prentice-Hall of Australia Pty., Limited, *Sydney*
Prentice-Hall Canada Inc., *Toronto*
Prentice-Hall Hispanoamericana, S.A., *Mexico*
Prentice-Hall of India Private Limited, *New Delhi*
Prentice-Hall of Japan, Inc., *Tokyo*
Simon & Schuster Asia Pte. Ltd., *Singapore*
Editora Prentice-Hall do Brasil, Ltda., *Rio de Janeiro*

Contents

3   General Pediatric Assessment   25

4   Equipment and Procedures for Management of ABCs   47

Preface

For more than a decade, the EMS community has continuously improved the care provided to children requiring emergency care. We recognize the federal initiative that provided the funding from the Department of Transportation (DOT), National Highway Traffic Safety Administration (NHTSA), and the Department of Health and Human Services, Bureau of Maternal and Child Health (DHHS, BMCH).

In 1983, Children's National Medical Center (CNMC) received funding from the Devore Foundation, Washington, D.C., to develop and offer a continuing medical education program for prehospital providers in pediatric emergency care. This experience led to the national Pediatric Emergency Medical Services Training Program (PEMSTP), funded by DOT and DHHS. This four-year project trained 190 EMS instructors from all 50 states, the District of Columbia, and two U.S. territories in pediatric emergency care. These instructors were encouraged to disseminate the pediatric knowledge and skills they learned back to their respective states.

The information contained in *Pediatric Emergencies* is the result of valuable experience we obtained while conducting prehospital education programs for EMS providers and instructors. These students shared their insights and suggestions to help shape the organization and content in this text, which is much more extensive than our first text, *Pediatric Emergencies Manual.*

The Emergency Medical and Trauma Services at CNMC recognizes the importance of prehospital care within its Continuum of Care philosophy. This continuum is initiated with Prevention activities, and includes organized care in the Prehospital, Emergency Department, Intensive Care Unit, General Care Unit, and Rehabilitation phases of care. The interdisciplinary nature of pediatric emergency care requires that both the prehospital and hospital team approach to the seriously ill or injured child be standardized and cohesive for an optimal outcome.

Pediatric Emergencies is written to document a standard of prehospital pediatric emergency care for both the basic and advanced levels of prehospital care providers. It is the intent of this text to convey that children are uniquely different from adults in anatomic, physiologic, and emotional characteristics that need special consideration when managing serious illness or injury.

The first chapters address the complex emotional and psychosocial characteristics of the child and family. The text identifies by developmental stage how each child deals with the fear of being in an emergency situation. The parents are equally anxious and may display a range of emotions that prehospital providers must recognize and manage. Having an understanding of the interdependent relationship between the parent and child enables the prehospital provider to better manage the child's care and to assist the child and family to work through their crisis.

Subsequent chapters of pediatric assessment and procedures for management of the ABCs are the keystones necessary in becoming proficient and confident in managing the pediatric patient. The assessment chapter gives the "how to" guidelines for approaching the child and the rationale. The descriptions of the anatomy and physiology identify the uniqueness of the child and justify the procedures discussed. The procedures chapter is thorough in explaining management strategies tailored to the pediatric patient. For example, because airway management is so important, significant attention is paid to all appropriate methods of basic and advanced life support airway management.

We have made every attempt to be comprehensive in presenting medical and trauma emergencies. Frequently encountered conditions, such as respiratory conditions and blunt trauma, are covered as well as those less frequently encountered, such as diabetic ketoacidosis and penetrating trauma. These chapters are organized with an overview of each condition, the physiologic responses of the child, assessment guidelines, and management. Both basic and advanced care is delineated to guide pediatric management for providers of different skill levels.

Several other chapters highlight the role of the prehospital provider in the emergency management of children. The newborn, small and unresisting, demands solid skill and knowledge to prevent rapid physiologic deterioration. The chapter on newborns focuses on the care of the infant after birth and safe transport to the hospital. Management of the newborn in distress is emphasized to ensure optimal care. Emergency care of the child with special needs due to a chronic health condition or terminal illness have also been addressed. There is a growing number of children with these conditions cared for at home assisted by high-technology equipment who may access EMS.

One concern addressed in the educational sessions conducted at CNMC was the feelings triggered in prehospital providers when managing the child and family in emergency situations. Feelings run strong when the prehospital provider sees his or her own child in the patient, confronts the injustice of child abuse or neglect, or relives the tragedy of a child's death. Dealing with parents who may be unreasonable and demanding adds another dimension to the duties of the prehospital provider, which can cause stress. For this reason, a chapter on stress recognition and management has been included.

In this second edition, the authors have attempted to keep in step with the changing National Curriculum for the prehospital provider. We remain impressed with the level of dedication, enthusiasm, and child advocacy that prehospital providers express in their quest for more knowledge about emergency care of children. We hope many of your current and future questions will be answered by this text.

Martin R. Eichelberger, M.D.
Jane W. Ball, R.N., Dr. P.H.
Geraldine L. Pratsch, R.N., M.P.H.
John R. Clark, NREMT-P

Acknowledgments

Without the overall vision of Senator Daniel K. Inouye, and the continuing efforts by his Administrative Assistant, Patrick H. DeLeon, Ph.D., the first and second editions of this book would not exist. The senator's vision for improved pediatric emergency care led to the development of the Pediatric Emergency Medical Services Training Program upon which this book was based. His continued sponsorship of the Emergency Medical Services for Children Program has allowed states to refine and implement training for prehospital providers so that children ultimately receive the needed child-specific emergency care.

The authors wish to thank Susan Katz, of Prentice Hall, for the opportunity to revise this textbook and for her support during this revision. Three prehospital provider instructors provided thoughtful comments and recommendations for the improvement of the manuscript, Patrick Malone, EMT-P, Andrew Stern, EMT-P, and Lisa Carlson, R.N., M.S. As with the first edition, George Dodson again helped broaden the visual appeal of the book with his sensitive photography of children and parents. We are also grateful to Silver Spring Ambulance Service who provided personnel and equipment for this edition's photography session. We are grateful to the parents, the children, and the Montgomery County, Maryland EMS providers who served as models for the first edition.

Ellie Runion, a coauthor of the first edition, was unable to continue collaboration with this edition. Her original contributions provided a strong foundation for several chapters in this revision. While she continues to be interested in the pediatric prehospital issues, she currently directs her energy as a child advocate within the hospital acute care system.

EMT instructors of the Pediatric Medical Services Training Program (PEMSTP) supported and encouraged the revision of this book, despite the extensive development of pediatric emergency resources developed through the Emergency Medical Services for Children Program. Mike McAdams, NREMT-P, a graduate of PEMSTP, must be acknowledged for his recommendations for the entire text revision and specifically the revision of the CPR chapter.

Finally, we must acknowledge and thank our families for their support during the revision of *Pediatric Emergencies*.

About the Authors

Martin R. Eichelberger, M.D., F.A.C.S., F.A.A.P., is Professor of Surgery and Pediatrics at the George Washington University School of Medicine and Director of the Emergency Medical and Trauma Services, Children's National Medical Center in Washington, D.C. His special interest in injured children led to the development of one of the nation's first pediatric trauma centers and the first pediatric emergency curriculum for prehospital providers. His particular interest in reducing the number of preventable injuries led to the initiation of the National SAFE KIDS Campaign in 1988 that now has coalitions in all 50 states. He served on the Institute of Medicine's National Panel that in 1993 made recommendations for improving the emergency medical services system for children. Author of many publications, he is also a research investigator on all aspects of care of the seriously ill or injured child, from prevention through pediatric trauma systems development to rehabilitation.

Jane W. Ball, R.N., Dr.P.H., is the Project Director of the Emergency Medical Services for Children National Resource Center based at Children's National Medical Center in Washington, D.C. In this role, she provides consultation and guidance to state health agencies and health professionals to improve pediatric emergency care systems. She also continues to serve as the program director of pediatric emergency education programs at the hospital. She previously served as the project coordinator of the Pediatric Emergency Medical Services Training Program, a nationwide federally funded project for instructors of prehospital providers. She also served as the project director of the Pediatric emergency Nursing Education Program, a federally funded project for emergency nurses in community hospitals of the mid-Atlantic region.

Geraldine L. Pratsch, R.N., M.P.H., is the Program Manager of the Emergency Medical and Trauma Services at the Children's National Medical Center in Washington, D.C. She previously served as the Pediatric Emergency Education Coordinator under the Devore Foundation grant project which evolved into the Pediatric Emergency Medical Services Training Program. She has been responsible for the development of regional and national prehospital education programs, workshops, and conferences. She is currently involved in the planning and modification of pediatric emergency and acute care delivery within the Emergency Medical Trauma Center to accommodate the changing health care environment.

John R. Clark, NREMT-P, is a Flight Paramedic with the PennSTAR Flight Program of the University of Pennsylvania Health System in Philadelphia, PA. He is a nationally registered paramedic with over 15 years experience in fire and rescue services. He served as the Education Coordinator for Prehospital Medicine at Children's National Medical Center in Washington, D.C., for 5 years, and he has used that experience to become a champion for issues and education related to prehospital pediatric care.

The Child's Response to Emergencies

OBJECTIVES

When you have completed this chapter you should be able to

▶ List and describe five stages of child development.
▶ List two primary concerns of a child at each developmental age group in an emergency situation.
▶ Identify three responses the emergency medical technician (EMT) can use with a child at each developmental age in an emergency situation.

Introduction

There is no way of knowing what is really going through a child's mind as he or she is taken away in an ambulance at the time of illness or injury. Seeing children in pain is difficult, especially when we have children of our own. We need to strike a balance among performing our duties in a professional manner, wishing to comfort the child, and identifying with the parents in their moment of helplessness, anxiety, and guilt.

Emergency medical technicians (EMTs) and paramedics need to be concerned with a child's emotional well-being, even during life-threatening events. A child that experiences such a frightening situation as being hit by a car and then having strangers touch him, apply equipment, and place him in an ambulance is vulnerable to emotional setbacks. Even under the best of circumstances (when the feelings of the child are taken into consideration and care for the physical illness or injury is successful), a child may experience regression, nightmares, and mistrust of adults.

When approaching the scene, remember a child's primary emotion is *fear* (Figure 1.1).

- Fear of being hurt and of having his or her body invaded and disfigured;
- Fear of being separated from the people and places that are familiar and of never returning home again;
- Fear of being in trouble for doing something wrong;
- Fear created by thoughts and images in the child's mind;
- Fear of the unknown.

The child will be distressed by the general air of panic and confusion that usually surrounds an emergency.

Prehospital treatment must be based on knowledge of the normal emotional and physiologic development of children. Well-intentioned treatment without the sufficient knowledge and skills in caring for a child's emotions places children and their families at unnecessary emotional risk.

FIGURE 1.1   The child's primary emotion is fear.

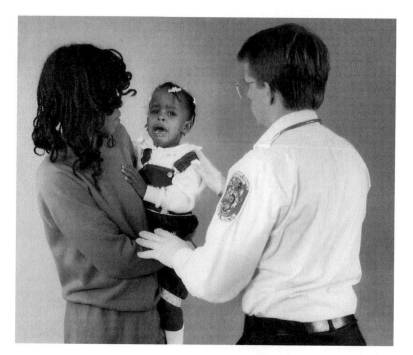

Chapter 1: The Child's Response to Emergencies

The Approach to the Child and Family

Rights of Children and Parents

Children and parents have a right to know what is being done and what to expect will be done to their bodies. For example, if the child is anxious and/or the parent is present, describe the treatment, directing it to the child in age-appropriate language. ("I need to put this long board under your leg to keep it from moving"). Avoid talking past the child by directing your instructions only to the parents. However, the language used for the child may not be appropriate for the parent. Avoid "talking down" to the parents. The parent/child relationship is extremely important to the child at this time, and children will seek consolation from parents. Do all that you can to provide for the child that parental emotional support (Figure 1.2).

Appropriate Language

Identify and use language of body parts that children will understand, such as *leg* and *tummy*. Avoid medical terms such as *femur* or *spleen*. Using unfamiliar terms will make both child and parent more anxious in an already tense situation.

Dealing with Pain

Always warn the child if a procedure or treatment will cause pain. Never say "This won't hurt" if it will. It is difficult to determine a child's level of pain, and thus the slightest movement of an extremity could trigger an outburst. If you know a procedure is going to hurt, have all equipment

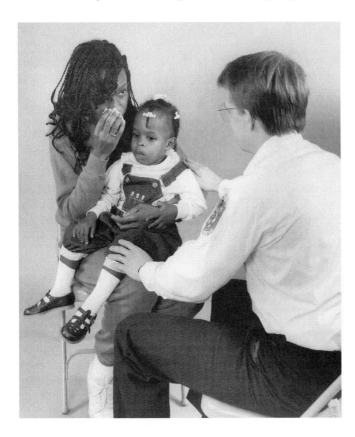

FIGURE 1.2 *"An injured child becomes an injured family." Remember to provide emotional support to the parent.*

ready, and then say, "Some children tell me this sometimes hurts. You tell me what it's like for you after we are done. Ready? . . . 1 . . . 2 . . . 3." Do not let the anticipation of pain build by allowing time between preparation for the procedure and doing it. After the procedure say, "I'm sorry that hurt."

Pain is very difficult for a preschool-age child to describe or localize. Ask, "What is the pain like—a sting, a scrape, or a mosquito bite?" School-age children may be able to describe the intensity of pain on a scale of 1–5 (5 being the worst pain ever felt and 1 being mild discomfort like a splinter). Ask the child to point to where the pain is to determine the location.

Avoid minimizing the hurt or intimidating the child by saying "That doesn't hurt" or "Big boys don't cry," or be a "brave boy" or "good girl." Sometimes the child seems too old chronologically to be crying and seems to be acting like a "baby." In this instance, deal with the behavior as it occurs. If a 10-year-old is acting like a 4-year-old, then treat that child as a 4-year-old. Remember, the child has no control over events, and crying is a coping mechanism.

Honesty

Be as honest as possible; however, use discretion. It is not necessary to tell the child that his or her mother is in critical condition and may not survive, or that the child's leg is severely damaged and he or she might lose it. Say, "I'm not sure what will happen. But I know what to do now to help you and get you to the doctors or hospital. Will you help me?"

When the child or parents ask you questions you cannot answer, do not feel obligated to give a reason or explanation. It is perfectly all right to say "I don't know." When the parent and child cannot be reassured that the child is all right, reassure them that everything possible is being done.

Sense of Hearing

Hearing is the last sense to go and first to return for the child slipping into unconsciousness or emerging from it. Therefore, assume the child can hear what is being said at all times. Talk to the child to reassure him or her, serving as a model for the parents. Even if the child is unconscious or hard to arouse, use the child's name when talking to him or her.

Emotional and Behavioral Development

An understanding of the emotional and behavioral development of infants and children is necessary for the EMT and paramedic to appropriately manage the child during prehospital care. As described in this chapter, the age breakdown is the accepted definition of infant, toddler, preschooler, etc., as commonly used and seen in the pediatric and growth-and-development literature.

Children with Special Health Care Needs

Children with special health care needs include children with a wide variety of health problems. Some children have physical disabilities, meaning they have trouble with movement or motor skills. Some children have cognitive disabilities, so that their ability to develop mentally is affected. Other children have social, communicative, and/or emotional problems. When working with these children, it is important to identify what the primary complaint is as well as any specific issues related to their disability.

Regardless of the child's abilities, each needs to be treated in a manner that is age-appropriate for the behavior exhibited (Figure 1.3).

Behavior at the Scene

Infant

The first year of life is one of rapid change. The newborn infant is physically and mentally immature and emotionally reacts at an instinctive level. The 12-month-old walks, talks, and exercises some independence, letting everyone know he or she has "arrived."

Birth to 6 Months

Young infants recognize the faces and voices of their parents and are emotionally tied to them. Infants experiencing pain in any portion of their body are unable to localize it. They have a whole-body response (crying, withdrawal, flexion of extremities) to any painful stimuli. This age group is physically easier to examine because infants are not very strong. On the other hand, because of small anatomic body parts, the infant's physiologic condition will deteriorate rapidly if not properly managed (Figure 1.4).

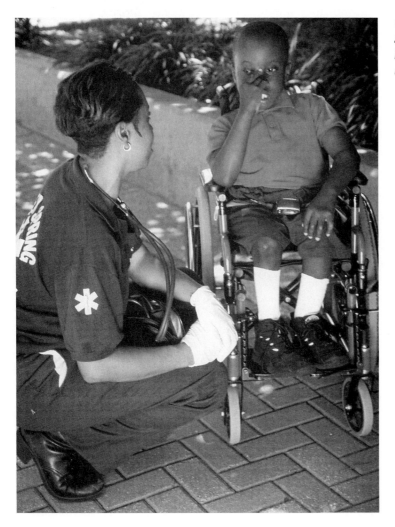

FIGURE 1.3 Treat a disabled child like all other children. Get down to his or her eye level to talk with the child and use age-appropriate language.

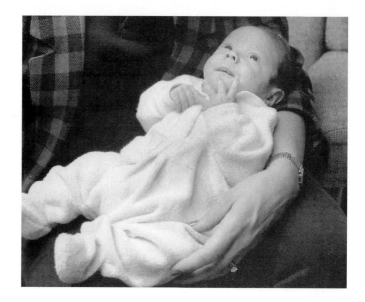

FIGURE 1.4 Infant less than 6 months.

6 to 12 Months

Older infants have a clear need of a parent or primary-care provider because they are very distressed by separation (Figure 1.5). They are not old enough to understand what is happening to them, and they resist being examined. If held in mother's arms, the infant will be more cooperative.

Your Approach at the Scene

Infants express emotional and physical distress through crying. Infants cope by seeking close physical contact with a parent or familiar person. If the condition permits, swaddle the younger infant in a blanket to provide a feeling of security. Allow the older infant to suck a thumb, pacifier, or bottle for comfort.

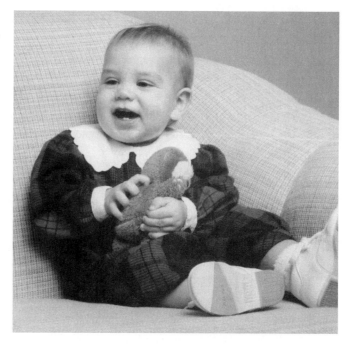

FIGURE 1.5 Infant greater than 6 months.

In emergencies, parents will be upset. Depending on the situation, be calm and reassure them that everything is going to be all right or that everything possible is being done. If you feel the parent will not interfere with treatment, let one parent ride in the back of the ambulance to provide a history and to comfort the infant. This may relieve some parental distress.

Prior to transport, examine the infant in the parent's arms or lap if there is no suspected cervical spine injury (Figure 1.6). Respect the child's "space." Do not rush to touch and examine the child without first observing the child's condition. Engage the parent in the examination. "I need to . . ., you can help me by . . ." Encourage parents to talk to, sing to, touch the infant (when appropriate) to reassure the infant and keep parents involved. (Refer to Chapter 3, "General Pediatric Assessment.")

Toddler

Development

Children between 1 and 3 years enjoy an age of intense activity and discovery. The toddler's philosophy of life is: Holes need to be filled up (including ears, nose, and mouth); everything needs to be touched, tasted, and manipulated; no one except a parent is to be trusted; nothing should be agreed to; and displeasure should be shown often and loudly (Figure 1.7).

Children 1 to 3 years of age are the most difficult to examine, even when they are not ill or injured. Problems are magnified by illness or injury. Toddlers will physically push you away, cry, scream, squirm, and do whatever is necessary to prevent you from touching them. Here you

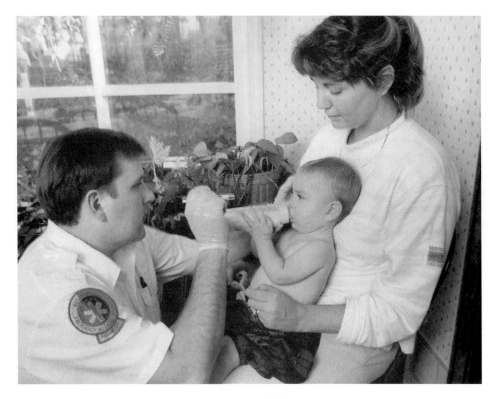

FIGURE 1.6 *Examining infant in mother's lap. Allow infant to suck a bottle for comfort during the examination.*

FIGURE 1.7
Toddler.

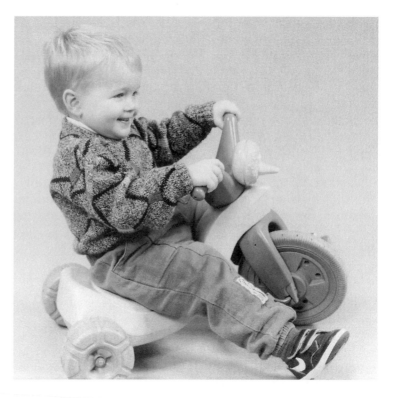

need to be flexible and take opportunities to perform the physical exam as the opportunity presents itself. This is where the *toe-to-head* assessment is the most beneficial, going from the less threatening parts of the body to the more threatening parts. In cases where the toddler is very uncooperative, concentrate on the component of the physical exam that is most important in obtaining information concerning the chief complaint. For example, if the child is having respiratory problems, concentrate on signs and symptoms of respiratory distress and level of consciousness and forego examination of the abdomen and extremities, etc.

Toddlers are the age group most likely to experience short-term and long-term emotional problems as a result of the emergency. Therefore, handle them with special care. Toddlers are terrified of separation from what is familiar, particularly the parent or primary-care provider. They do not understand that things are being done for their benefit. They have limited language skills and thus have difficulty understanding verbal explanations.

The toddler's biggest fear is the possibility of separation from the parent or that which is familiar, such as a toy or stuffed animal. Fear of strangers is also strongly expressed. The toddler copes by seeking physical contact with the parent. A dependency object such as toy, stuffed animal, or blanket is often used by the toddler for a feeling of security.

Your Approach at the Scene

Talk to the child in a reassuring and quiet tone of voice, repeating a phrase such as "I'm here to help you." Tone of voice conveys reassurance even though the child may not understand your words. If restraining the child is needed, be as gentle as possible. When necessary, human restraints are preferable to mechanical ones. Be sure the child has a toy, stuffed animal, or other dependency object alongside while being transported in the ambulance (Figure 1.8). Some rescue units have a stuffed animal on board to distract the child or use it to help with the examination. If a

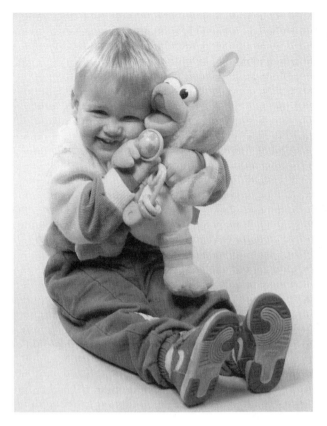

FIGURE 1.8 *Toddler with dependency objects.*

stuffed animal is given to the child it may be problematic in retrieving it at the end of the run. In this instance, repossessing it seems inappropriate. Keep the parent nearby; allow the parent to touch or hold the child so as to calm him or her and to incorporate the parent as part of the exam or have the parent assist during the examination.

Preschooler

Development

During the preschool period (3 to 5 years of age), basic skills such as walking, running, talking, toilet training, etc., have been accomplished and are being refined. Running, once an enjoyment within itself, is now a means to a bigger and better end. This child has full awareness of the external body and body parts. Concrete thinking and literal interpretation of what is heard is normal. The preschooler has a vivid imagination and can dramatize events (Figure 1.9).

Preschoolers are likely to believe an accident or injury is their fault, regardless of whether or not they had a role in bringing it about. While they have better verbal skills, they do not have complex language skills and can misinterpret common words. They do not understand their internal anatomy. Preschoolers continue to have the fears of younger children, particularly of separation and abandonment. Use of the *toe-to-head* approach for the assessment is also appropriate for these children, depending on the circumstances and age of the child.

Preschoolers are very frightened of physical injury and especially the sight of blood on their body. Fears related to body integrity such as mutilation or body intactness are intense. Band-Aids help in covering the wound so that the child can avoid looking at it.

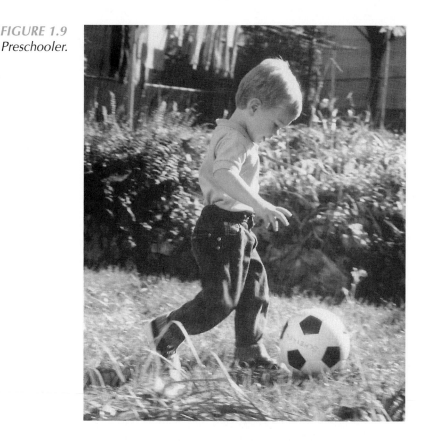

FIGURE 1.9
Preschooler.

When coping with pain, the preschooler's need for the parent is still great, especially the young preschooler. Oftentimes they regress to a younger stage of behavior, crying or resisting examination and care.

Your Approach at the Scene

Approach the child slowly. Do not stand over the child—try to get down to their level. These children might appear to understand what is occurring when actually they do not. Be certain that your reassuring and quiet tone of voice gets through to the child, even if nothing else does. Employ the toe-to-head assessment if appropriate.

Use simple words to describe the care to be given; do this for the benefit of both the parent and the child. Let the child know it is okay to cry. If there is a visible injury, particularly a bloody one, clean it and dress it (Figure 1.10). Blood in the eyes from a scalp wound can be far more terrifying to children than the extent of the injury suggests to you.

School Age

Development

The 6-to-12-year age group covers a wide range of differing levels of behavior and development. During these middle childhood years, the child learns and develops through games, contacts with peers, relationships with family, and the environment of home, school, and community (Figure 1.11).

School-age children can understand rational explanations and are probably the easiest to examine and manage. However, they are still frightened and may see illness or injury as a punishment. The school-age child fears pain, punishment, and separation from family and friends. While

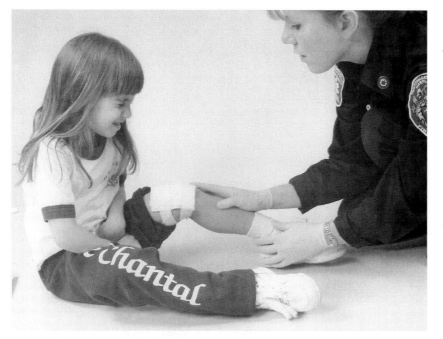

FIGURE 1.10 Cover the injury to reduce the child's anxiety.

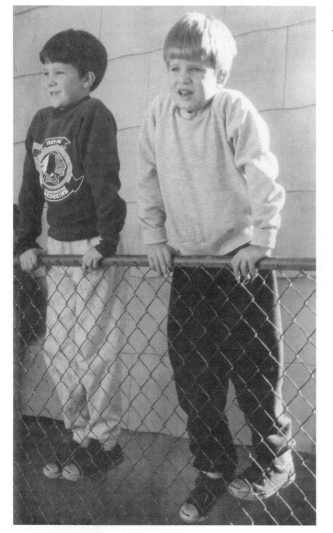

FIGURE 1.11
School-age children.

these children do not understand technical words, they have simple understanding of internal anatomy. Issues of modesty are very important, and these children do not like their bodies exposed to strangers. Concerns about death and disability emerge during this stage of development.

Early school-age children may regress under stress of an emergency. Parents are needed to validate the child's reactions to the illness or injury in order to help the child adjust. How the parents cope will influence how the child copes.

Your Approach at the Scene

Include the child in conversation, particularly when obtaining the history. Direct the history questions to the child and explain in simple terms what you are doing during examination and treatment. If you wish to understand their level of knowledge of what is happening, ask questions in the third party, such as "Do you know other people who went to the hospital? What happened to them? What do you think will happen to you?"

The *head-to-toe* assessment is appropriate with these children. The parent will appropriately respond to history questions and appreciate the explanation of care. Do not belittle the child's pain or threaten or trick the child who protests. This will help reassure both child and parent that everything possible is being done. Make every attempt to cover the child's body so that it is not exposed excessively (Figure 1.12).

This child will be interested in what is in the ambulance. Explain the function of the equipment and indicate that not all pieces of equipment will be used on him or her. To the best of your ability, prepare the child for what is going to be done at the hospital. "When you arrive at the hospital, there will be lots of doctors and nurses. They will listen to your heart and measure your blood pressure like I did, then. . . ."

FIGURE 1.12 *Expose only the portion of the child's body that needs to be examined.*

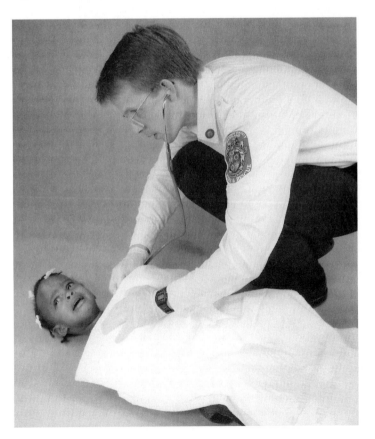

Chapter 1: The Child's Response to Emergencies

Adolescent

Development

The period between 13 and 18 years is an age of many changes and decisions as the adolescent leaves childhood and enters the world of the young adult in search of independence. Because adolescents possess concrete thinking and are developing abstract thinking, they can deal with the present and project into the future. The adolescent has incredible drive and energy and commonly engages in "magical thinking" with feelings of indestructibility (Figure 1.13).

Adolescents generally understand what is happening and are often the best historians. On the other hand, adolescents are tremendously preoccupied with their bodies even when not threatened by illness or injury. These concerns are intensified when there is bodily injury. They fear permanent disability or disfigurement and they are aware of the possibility of their own death. Modesty is a very real issue with this group. Personal clothing can be very important to an adolescent.

Adolescents of both sexes are capable of a "hysterical" reaction to illness or injury, which often impresses outsiders as "overdoing" it. Instances of "mass hysteria" may be observed in adolescents, as when a great number of children seem to suffer food poisoning or are overcome by fumes, etc. Generally, even "hysterical" adolescents respond to quiet reassurance.

Your Approach at the Scene

Try to have the assessment of the adolescent done by someone of the same sex (Figure 1.14). In all cases, respect the teenager's feelings of modesty. Reassure the adolescent that he or she is not going to die (even if you feel that is possible). Instead, say that "We are doing everything we can as fast as possible to get you to the hospital for the care you need." If the adolescent appears "hysterical" and seems to be overreacting, be tolerant of

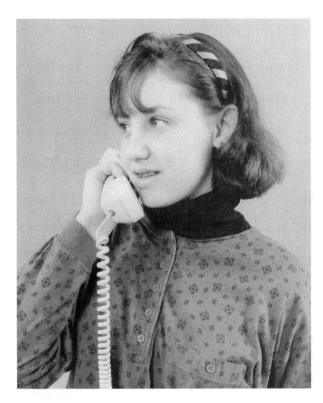

FIGURE 1.13 Adolescent.

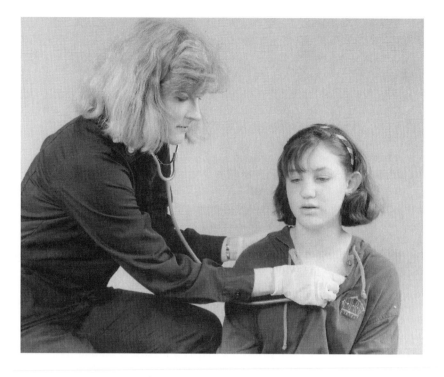

FIGURE 1.14   Try to provide assessment of the adolescent by an EMT of the same sex.

this; do not get caught up in the hysteria or become angry about it. In most cases, the parents do not need to accompany the teenager in the ambulance. Explain to the adolescent what is happening and what will probably happen at the hospital. Talk directly to the adolescent, not around him or her to the parent. Consider confidentiality. Questions about sex or drugs need to be discreet.

The Child's Response References

Brennan, A., "Caring for children during procedures: A review of the literature," *Pediatric Nursing,* 20, no. 5 (September/October 1994), pp. 451–458.

Davenport, L.B., "Life-threatening situations: Supporting the child and family," *Journal of Pediatric Nursing,* 10, no. 4 (August 1995), pp. 219–223.

Duncan, C.M., "Kids are patients too," *Emergency,* 26, no. 8 (August 1994), pp. 34–39.

Gatz, R.R., "Children's responses to emergency department care," *Annals of Emergency Medicine,* 13, no. 5 (May 1984), pp. 322–333.

_____ . "What makes kids sick: Children's beliefs about causative factors of illness," *Children's Health Care,* 12 (Spring 1984), pp. 157–162.

Grover, G., "Talking to children." In Berkowitz, C.D., ed., *Pediatrics: A Primary Approach.* Philadelphia: W.B. Saunders Co., 1996, pp. 7–9.

Kemp, V., "The relationship of temperament and children's crying behavior during a stressful situation," *Children's Health Care,* 13, no. 2 (1984), pp. 59–63.

Pontious, S.L., "Practical Piaget: Helping children understand," *American Journal of Nursing,* 82, no. 1 (January 1982), pp. 114–117.

Reynolds, E.A., and Ramenofsky, M.L., "Emotional impact of trauma on toddlers," *Maternal Child Nursing,* 13, (March/April 1988), pp. 106–109.

Robinson, C.A., "Preschool children's conceptualizations of health and illness," *Children's Health Care,* 16, no. 2 (Fall 1987), pp. 89–95.

Sifuentes, M., "Talking to adolescents." In Berkowitz, C.D., ed., *Pediatrics: A Primary Care Approach.* Philadelphia: W.B. Saunders Co., 1996, pp. 10–12.

Family Members' Response to Their Child's Emergency

OBJECTIVES

When you have completed this chapter you should be able to

▶ Describe three types of reactions or emotions exhibited by parents in an emergency involving their child.
▶ Describe three different methods for dealing with the family in a pediatric emergency.

Pediatric professionals who care for children realize that treating the child requires treating the family as well. When the child experiences discomfort and pain with illness or injury, the parents suffer almost equally with anxiety and emotional stress.

In an emergency, the parents' reaction to the child's emergency condition is "acute anxiety." This is a normal reaction to a distressing situation manifested by psychological and somatic symptoms. The range of emotions associated with the anxiety expressed by parents includes fear, shock, denial, guilt, anger, and loss of control. Whatever behavior the parent is demonstrating when you arrive at the scene is the way that particular parent is managing anxiety *at that particular time*. Parents' behavior may, however, change dramatically during the time prehospital care is provided (Figure 2.1).

The most common parental reaction noted by EMTs and paramedics is having no control over the situation. Relinquishing their child to your care, not knowing what will happen next, and worrying about the child's condition leave parents feeling helpless. Because of this, parents may ask questions such as:

- "Is my child going to die?"
- "Will he be OK?"
- "Is his brain OK?"
- "Will he walk again?"

FIGURE 2.1   Parents display a range of emotions in response to their child's emergency condition.

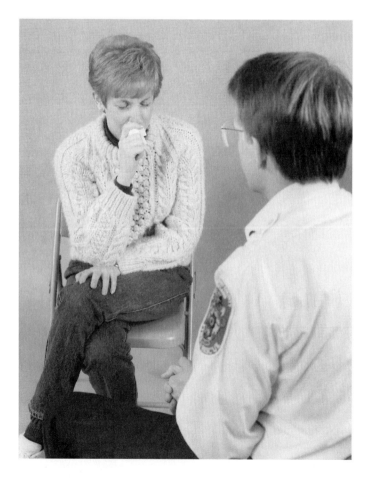

Parents in emotional shock respond differently. They are pale, quiet, and uncommunicative; they are withdrawn, stare into space, and may be unaware of another presence. They may not respond or be slow to respond to your questions.

Sometimes parents become very demanding in an attempt to control the situation and help their child. This can be a very uncomfortable situation for the EMT. Sometimes these parents may get in your way, preventing you from doing your job effectively.

When responding to a pediatric emergency, the EMT should respond to the parent in the following ways:

■ Acknowledge the feelings of the parent. "This must be very upsetting to you."
■ Reassure the parent that "it's understandable to feel the way you do."
■ Redirect the parents' energies to help you in some way in caring for their child. "I could really use your help."
■ Remain calm and appear in control to help parents deal with their anxiety. Try not to raise your voice or become antagonistic.
■ Project confidence to family members so they trust you and believe everything possible is being done to stabilize the child's condition and to provide transport as soon as possible to the hospital.
■ Provide additional information as necessary.
■ Answer questions appropriately.

Guidelines for Verbal and Nonverbal Communication with Parents

Set the Tone During the Rescue

■ Be calm
■ Introduce yourself and identify your job responsibilities.
■ Call the child by name; also use the surname of the parent. For example, "Mrs. Blake, we will be taking Jimmy to the trauma center at Children's Hospital."
■ Be supportive and nonjudgmental.

Remember That Your First Priority Is to the Ill or Injured Child

■ Help family members with their crisis without compromising patient care. Patient care is your main objective and responsibility, and it should never be compromised. However, dealing with the parents is a fact of life, and this chapter will assist you in coping with parental reactions to a child in crisis.
■ Initiate your assessment in an efficient and rapid manner. Parents are reassured when their child is cared for by professionals who take their work seriously and who project a concerned, caring, and competent attitude.
■ Consider having the parents be helpers or go-betweens in communicating with the child. They can help to keep the child calm.

Keep Calm: You Are in a Crisis-Management Situation

- Through all of this, the one positive image that you must project is that of competence and caring. That in turn will foster trust.
- Keep calm, even though you may be apprehensive about the situation.
- Project an image that everything possible is being done and the best possible care is being delivered so as to ease anxious family members. Professionalism is important to gain the trust of the parents.

Keep the Parents Informed and Keep the Language Simple

- Anticipate what type of information parents want and need to know during each step of the assessment (Figure 2.2).
- Explain as you proceed with the examination and treatment or give a short synopsis of the overall condition of the child. For example: "I'm feeling Susie's abdomen for any internal bumps or bruises" or "The blood on Tim's head is from a cut; it will probably need some stitches. We have a bandage on the wound to stop the bleeding until we get to the emergency room." The responses you get to this type of interaction help you determine how the parents are handling the situation and how to assist them.

If you have difficulty controlling a parent, seek assistance from another family member or another professional (prehospital provider or police).

Ask for the Parents' Assistance

- The parent and child should not be separated unless the parent is totally out of control and interfering with your care.
- Ask parents who are capable, "Would you hold his [her] hands while I look at his [her] chest and abdomen?" (Figure 2.3)

FIGURE 2.2   Provide information to parent.

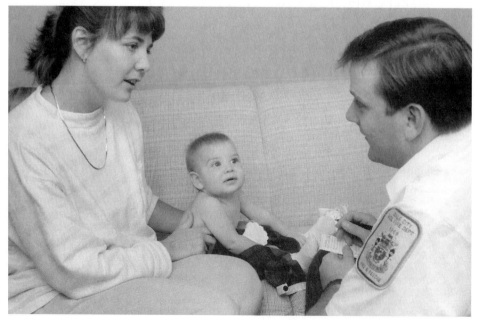

Chapter 2: Family Members' Response to Their Child's Emergency

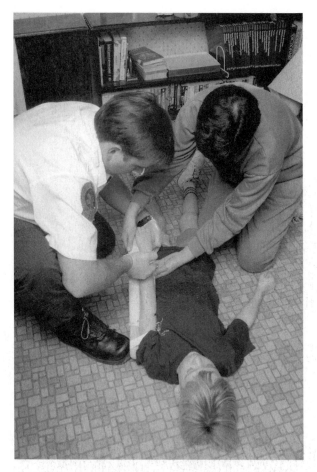

FIGURE 2.3   Enlist parents' help as you assess or treat their child.

- If the child is seriously injured, ask, "Would you please stand here? I may need your help." Try to make the parents feel they are participating in the care given to their child, even if it is only by asking questions or providing the history.

Be Honest with the Parent and Child

- If you must perform a procedure that is particularly painful for the child, explain what needs to be done and the reason. For example: "Billy, I'm going to put your leg in this splint and it's going to hurt for a short time. The splint prevents further injury to your leg until we get to the hospital. While I'm doing that, I want you to squeeze your Dad's hand as hard as you can, and it's okay to cry."

Provide Parents with Some Words of Reassurance About Their Child's Condition

- Emphasize the positive. "Your child is breathing fine. His blood pressure is good. He may have a broken leg, but he has good toe movement and good pulses in the foot."
- Avoid giving the parents *false* reassurances with such phrases as "Sam will be fine" if that is not the case. You may be promising more than the best medical care can deliver.

Guidelines for Verbal and Nonverbal Communication with Parents

- If the situation is grave and the parents ask, "Is she going to die?" tell them, "I don't know; we're going to do our best for your daughter." With that statement, you are being honest and preparing them for the potential loss (Figure 2.4).

At many hospitals, professionals are available to help parents deal with their child's serious condition or death and to begin the grieving process.

Do Not Show Family Members or Bystanders Your Personal Negative Feelings Concerning the Circumstances at the Scene

- As a professional in a position of authority, your initial reaction sets the tone of how the parents will respond and cooperate with the treatment of their child from the scene through hospital care. Try to be as nonjudgmental as possible.
- If you reveal your negative feelings, family members may either panic and try to interfere with treatment or assume additional

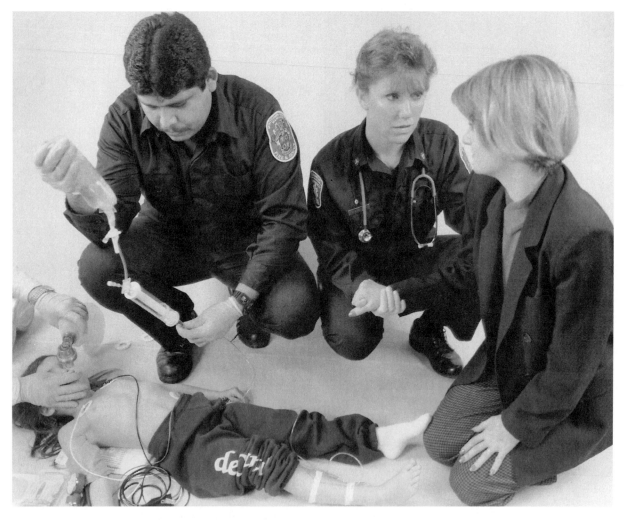

FIGURE 2.4 *Showing concern for the parent during treatment of the child.*

Chapter 2: Family Members' Response to Their Child's Emergency

unwarranted guilt. Many parents blame themselves for any serious illness or injury of their child, whether or not they were responsible. If they feel that you or other professionals blame them for what happened to their child, their psychological adjustments may be more difficult.

- For example, situations where the gate was left unlocked or the household cleaning agent was left within reach should be evaluated objectively, without verbal or nonverbal judgment. When abuse or neglect is suspected, refer this information to the appropriate hospital personnel, community social service agency, or law enforcement agency.
- Even when abuse is suspected, the parent and child should be transported together. These children have the same fears of separation from parents as do other children. (See Chapter 13, "Child Abuse.")

Show Concern for the Family Members During the Process of Management and Transport

- When people panic, it is difficult for them to organize effectively. Remind parents to lock their doors, turn off the stove, bring a coat or their wallet, and make arrangements with neighbors to look after their other children.
- Have a parent ride in the ambulance if appropriate.
- If the child is to be transported by helicopter, assess the parent's ability to drive to the hospital. If possible, find a friend, neighbor, or police to transport them. If they drive themselves, remind them to drive safely and not to try to keep up with the ambulance. Tell them to obey all traffic laws and say you will meet them at the hospital.
- Be sure the parent knows the name, location, and phone number of the hospital where you are taking the child. Make sure someone has directions if it is distant.
- When at the hospital, show them where to sit, offer tissues, and let them know the next step. Introduce them to the staff taking over. Before you leave say goodbye and offer words of encouragement. Any act of kindness will be remembered.

Accept the Parents' Reaction to the Situation

- Whether the parents are angry, hysterical, or in shock, they are doing the best they can in this very trying and unreal situation. Your nonjudgmental attitude affords them permission to start working through their fears and anxiety to face reality.

What About the Feelings of the Prehospital Care Provider?

- After you have had a particularly difficult situation involving a child, talk to someone you trust about it. Talking to a colleague, partner, hospital staff member, or unit supervisor may help you cope with the very difficult work that you are asked to perform. (See Chapter 17, "Crisis and Stress Management," for additional details.)

Table 2.1 lists some of the common reactions that parents have in an emergency involving their child and offers examples of EMT interventions.

TABLE 2.1 ■ *Common Parental Reactions to Sudden, Life-Threatening Conditions*

PARENTAL BEHAVIOR DURING FIRST IMPACT OF CRISIS	REASONS FOR THE BEHAVIOR	SUGGESTED RESPONSES
Shock or Denial		
Parents may be in a daze and seem incapable of absorbing the reality of the illness/injury.	Sometimes it is too difficult to integrate the loss or potential loss of the child into the conscious process of the mind.	Do not force the parent to face reality. Remain calm, use simple but direct explanations, and offer reassurance and support. Write things down for them. Repeat information at a later time.
The "numb" reaction makes it difficult to understand explanations about the situation.	Numbness enables the parent to *slowly* begin to feel the impact of the seriousness of the situation.	Parents in denial sometimes do not hear the assessment information being told to them. Keep the parent informed concerning the child's condition and the need for transport. They may try to get you to say that everything will be okay.
Parents in a state of denial react by saying, "I don't believe it." "He was fine when I put him to bed." "There must be a mistake." "I know he will be fine."	Denial is a normal mechanism of trying to keep the terrible truth from hitting all at once.	
Parents may be overly compliant or "matter of fact."	Parents are distancing themselves to protect themselves from being emotionally overwhelmed.	The appearance of having themselves under control may be a facade, and they could break down at any moment.
Crying, Screaming, Intense Rage, and Bitterness		
Some parents react immediately with an intense emotional display to the potential loss of the child or the potential loss of normal functioning.	The suddenness and severity of the illness or injury may make it impossible for the parent to use denial as a defense. Anger helps the parents from being overwhelmed.	You may feel uncomfortable with the parents openly expressing such intense feelings. Don't discourage them. Do listen, give information, and provide reassurance. Extreme behavior may need police intervention.
Some will lash out at God, the spouse, the sibling, the school, the baby-sitter, the driver of the other vehicle, the doctor who didn't find anything wrong last week, etc. Some will cry out and remain in one place; others will be agitated and pace the floor, slam their fists into walls, or physically lash out at those rendering care.	Crying openly and intensely is a common way of dealing with tragedy. In some cases parents may be displaying what could be interpreted as overreacting, when in reality the parent may be getting ready for the worst.	Often, parents become embarrassed about their open expressions of sorrow, rage, etc. Reassure them that such expressions are normal under the circumstances. Let them know that other parents react this way then their child's life is threatened. Acknowledge the feelings but say they need to pull themselves together to help their child.
Expressions of Guilt and Self-Blame by the Parent		
In the event of sudden illness, the parent may blame himself or herself for "not paying enough attention to the sore throat or fever"—"for canceling last week's checkup"—"for not giving enough cough medicine," etc. If the child is injured, the parent will often blame himself or herself for "letting him ride his bicycle,"—"for crossing the busy street,"—"for driving too fast,"—"for letting him play football," etc. If the anger was expressed (or felt), the parent may be feeling very guilty.	Parents look for a "reason" for the catastrophe. It is easier to blame something than to accept the current event. If one could figure out why something happened, one could keep it from happening again. Some guilt may have deep roots. Some guilt has to do with recent events in which something unpleasant occurred to strain the parent-child relationship.	Listen to the parents' anguish. Let them verbalize their thoughts. If the parent says, "My teenager said that I should go to work—that he would stay in bed and would be fine," and the mother found him to be unconscious when she came home, reassure the mother that she made the best decision she could at the time. Generally, teenagers who get sick do fine with some rest. No one can blame the mother for going to work. Most parents would have done the same thing under the circumstances. There was no way to anticipate or protect the child from this event.

Chapter 2: Family Members' Response to Their Child's Emergency

TABLE 2.1 ■ *Common Parental Reactions to Sudden, Life-Threatening Conditions (cont.)*

PARENTAL BEHAVIOR DURING FIRST IMPACT OF CRISIS	REASONS FOR THE BEHAVIOR	SUGGESTED RESPONSES
Controlling Hysterical Behavior Toward the EMT		
Parents may become so agitated that they interfere with the examination and treatment of their child. They tell the EMTs that they (the EMTs) do not know what they are doing—that the child should not be treated at the scene, that the procedures are worthless, etc.	Parents feel it is their role to protect their children from all threats. In most instances, it is healthy for parents to try to exert "some" control over events in the life of the child.	In most instances, the parents' need to control may work to the advantage of the EMT. Help channel their energy in a more positive way. Have the parent hold the child's hand, comfort the child, accompany the child to the hospital, provide a good medical history, help explain why certain procedures must be carried out, etc.
In some instances, parents may exert physical control over the EMT. It is the response to the adrenaline surge of "fight or flight."	It is an innate response of some parents to physically protect children from perceived harm.	However, if the parent is out of control and interferes with the care of the child, the EMT must get help from a relative, friends, police, etc. This makes it possible to restrain and comfort the parent or to run interference to allow the EMT to perform necessary procedures on the child.

The Family's Response References

Back, K.J., "Sudden, unexpected pediatric death: Caring for the parents," *Pediatric Nursing*, 17, no. 6 (November/December 1991), pp. 571–575.

Davenport, L.B., "Life-threatening situations: Supporting the child survivor and the family," *Journal of Pediatric Nursing*, 10, no. 4 (August 1995), pp. 219–223.

Gibbons, M.B., "Listening to the lived experience of loss," *Pediatric Nursing*, 19, no. 6 (November/December 1993), pp. 597–599.

McIntier, T.M., "Nursing the family when a child dies," *RN*, 58 (February, 1995), pp. 50–54.

Miles, A., "Caring for families when a child dies," *Pediatric Nursing*, 16, no. 4 (July/August 1990), pp. 346–347.

Steward, E.S., "Family-centered care for the bereaved," *Pediatric Nursing*, 21, no. 2 (March/April 1995), pp. 181–194.

General Pediatric Assessment

OBJECTIVES

When you have completed this chapter you should be able to

▶ Identify one anatomic or physiologic difference between children and adults for each of the following areas:
- Skin and body surface area
- Head
- Airway
- Chest
- Abdomen
- Blood volume

▶ List approaches to improve the child's cooperation during the physical examination.

▶ Identify four areas to consider when taking the child's history.

▶ Identify important observations to make about the child's appearance and condition before touching the child.

▶ Describe important factors in taking and interpreting each of the following vital signs:
- Pulse
- Respirations
- Blood pressure
- Temperature

To interpret the findings from a physical examination of infants and children, it is important to understand the differences in anatomy and physiology between children and adults. Most special features of the child's anatomy and physiology are directly related to their smaller size and the continual growth and development of body systems. See Figure 3.1 for an overview of the unique anatomic and physiologic features of infants and young children.

Skin and Body Surface Area

Children's body or **skin surface area** is proportionately larger for their weight than an adult's. The head of an infant or young child accounts for approximately 20% of the total body surface area, and is larger and heavier in comparison to the rest of the body, until about 4 years of age. Proportions of body surface area by body part change throughout childhood, assuming adult dimensions by about 10 years of age. (See Figure 12.3, page 185.)

The skin of both infants and young children is thinner and more delicate, containing less subcutaneous fat, than an adult's. The same exposure to burn injury will result in deeper burns than what adults receive.

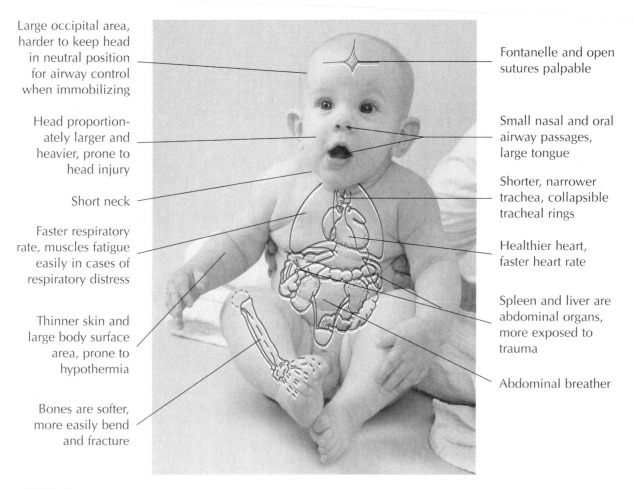

Large occipital area, harder to keep head in neutral position for airway control when immobilizing

Head proportionately larger and heavier, prone to head injury

Short neck

Faster respiratory rate, muscles fatigue easily in cases of respiratory distress

Thinner skin and large body surface area, prone to hypothermia

Bones are softer, more easily bend and fracture

Fontanelle and open sutures palpable

Small nasal and oral airway passages, large tongue

Shorter, narrower trachea, collapsible tracheal rings

Healthier heart, faster heart rate

Spleen and liver are abdominal organs, more exposed to trauma

Abdominal breather

FIGURE 3.1   *The unique anatomic and physiologic features of infants and young children.*

The large surface area for body mass and thinner layer of subcutaneous fat contribute to problems in maintaining body temperature. For this reason, children are more prone to develop *hypothermia.* Newborns are at even greater risk because their body temperature regulatory mechanisms are not well developed. Infants and children should be kept warm with minimal exposure to the environment. Covering the head is especially important for infants to help them stay warm. Resuscitation efforts and drug therapies are not as effective in a hypothermic child.

Head

The bones of the skull are soft and separated by cartilage until about 5 years of age. The cartilage suture lines permit growth and expansion of the skull as the brain grows. Because the skull is expandable, the child may be able to survive increased intracranial pressure for a *short* time without major complications.

Fontanelles are diamond-shaped soft spots of fibrous tissue found at the top of the skull where three or four individual bones will eventually fuse together. This fibrous tissue is very strong, and in normal circumstances it adequately protects the brain from injury. The anterior fontanelle closes (is covered by bone) between 12 and 18 months of age, and the posterior fontanelle closes by 2 months of age (Figure 3.2).

All of the brain cells a person will ever have are present at birth; however, they are not fully developed. Neurologic development proceeds over several years as the brain cells grow in size and nerve endings develop and connect. Brain cell development is complete by 5 years of age. Motor development proceeds from the head to the trunk and distally to the extremities as nerve connections develop. For this reason, head control develops before an infant can sit or walk.

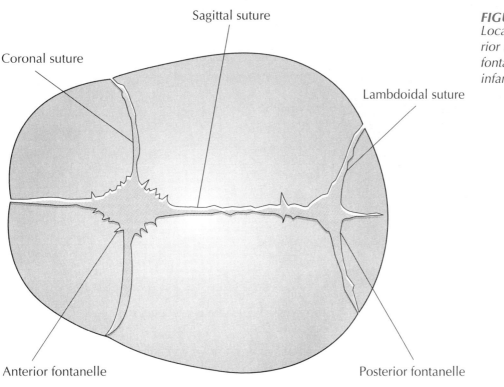

Sagittal suture

Coronal suture

Lambdoidal suture

Anterior fontanelle

Posterior fontanelle

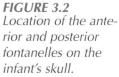

FIGURE 3.2
Location of the anterior and posterior fontanelles on the infant's skull.

The developing brain of an infant or young child is sensitive to poisons, infections, and injury, which may result in major neurologic defects and permanent disabilities. The brain tissue is thinner, softer, and more flexible than an adult's. The *dura*, the tissue surrounding the brain, is firmly attached to the skull in children and is more likely to be torn away with injury and result in bleeding into subdural spaces.

Airway

The face of the young child is smaller than an adult's but not necessarily small in proportion to head size. The nasal bridge is flat and flexible. Face masks must be selected for a proper size and shape to obtain a good seal.

Nasal passages are small in diameter, becoming easily obstructed with foreign objects or secretions. Newborns and young infants are obligate nose breathers, meaning they do not automatically open the mouth to breathe when the nose becomes obstructed. They will develop respiratory distress if nasal passages become obstructed. See Figure 3.3 for illustration of the airway characteristics.

The child's tongue is large in comparison to the size of the mouth. Pressure on the soft tissues under the chin can easily press the tongue to the back of the mouth and cause an airway obstruction. The muscles controlling the jaw are immature, permitting the mandible to fall back toward the throat and the tongue to obstruct the airway when the child is supine. For these reasons, the tongue is the major cause of airway obstruction in children.

The size of the trachea is small in comparison to an adult's; thus, any inflammation or swelling in the airway seriously compromises ventilation (Figure 3.4).

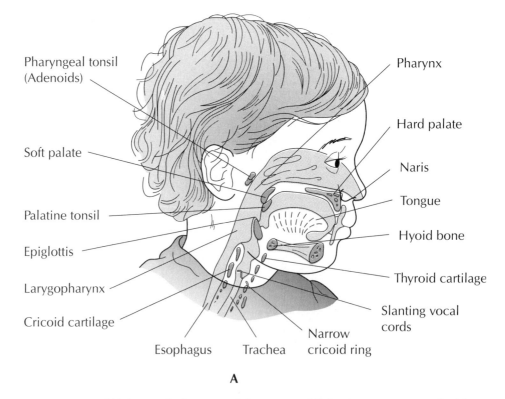

Pharyngeal tonsil (Adenoids)

Soft palate

Palatine tonsil

Epiglottis

Larygopharynx

Cricoid cartilage

Esophagus   Trachea   Narrow cricoid ring

Pharynx

Hard palate

Naris

Tongue

Hyoid bone

Thyroid cartilage

Slanting vocal cords

A

FIGURE 3.3   *(A) Anatomic features of the young child's airway, contrasted with that of (B) the adult's airway.*

- The diameter of the trachea is approximately 4 mm in an infant (about the diameter of a drinking straw) compared to 20 mm in an adult. The smallest tracheal diameter is in the subglottic area at the cricoid (until about age 8) rather than at the cords.
- The length of the trachea is 4 to 5 cm in a newborn and 7 cm by 18 months; this compares to 12 cm in an adult.

The tracheal cartilage rings are more elastic in children and collapse easily. Hyperextension or flexion of the child's neck can crimp the trachea, leading to an airway obstruction.

The larynx is higher and more anterior in the child, at the level of the 3rd or 4th cervical vertebrae, compared to the 5th or 6th cervical vertebrae in the adult. The epiglottis is higher, often visible when looking in the mouth. This high position contributes to aspiration by the child, especially if the neck is hyperextended. The epiglottic folds are more elastic and interfere with visualization of the vocal cords during intubation. Neutral or "sniffing" position is the best for managing the child's airway.

Chest and Lungs

The rib cage of both infant and young child is more elastic and flexible as it is composed of more cartilage than bone. Rib fractures are less common in children; this is because the force of injury is dissipated over the chest. Lung tissue is fragile, and pulmonary contusion is the most common result of a thoracic injury. In addition, the child has a mobile mediastinum, meaning the heart and large blood vessels can shift position, leading to a greater tendency to develop a tension pneumothorax.

Chest muscles are not well developed in children, and the diaphragm is the primary muscle for ventilatory effort. The healthy child will have minimal chest movement with respirations; however, the abdomen should rise with inspiration and fall with expiration. Chest muscles are accessory respiratory muscles in the young child, used in cases of respiratory distress.

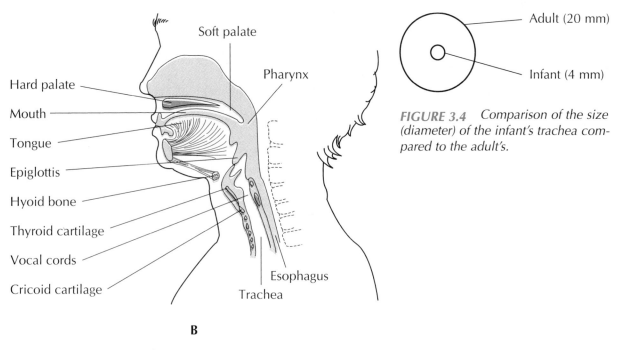

Hard palate

Mouth

Tongue

Epiglottis

Hyoid bone

Thyroid cartilage

Vocal cords

Cricoid cartilage

Soft palate

Pharynx

Esophagus

Trachea

B

Adult (20 mm)

Infant (4 mm)

FIGURE 3.4   Comparison of the size (diameter) of the infant's trachea compared to the adult's.

FIGURE 3.3   (Continued)

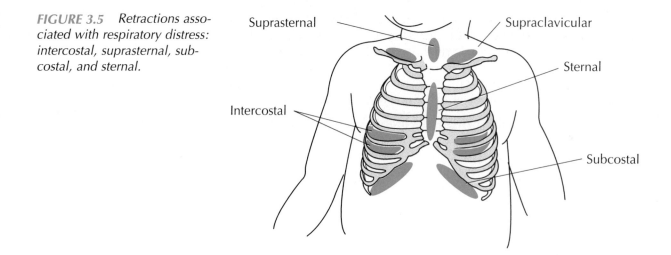

FIGURE 3.5 Retractions associated with respiratory distress: intercostal, suprasternal, subcostal, and sternal.

Retractions are the result of the flexible rig cage and use of accessory muscles for breathing. Intercostal retractions (between the ribs) are seen with mild respiratory distress. Sternal (sternum sinking on inspiration), suprasternal (above the sternum), and supraclavicular (in the neck above the clavicles) retractions are seen as respiratory distress progresses in severity (Figure 3.5).

Normal respiratory rates vary with age; the younger the child, the faster the rate (Table 3.1). Stress of any kind (fear, fever, excitement) will stimulate an increase in the child's respiratory rate. This hyperventilation may lead to gastric dilation. Hypoxia results in a progressively more rapid respiratory rate if not treated with oxygen.

■ Breathing becomes ineffective at rates faster than 60 breaths per minute in children. Air moves only in the upper airway, never reaching the lungs, when hyperventilation occurs. This leads to respiratory failure if not managed properly.

■ Children have immature chest muscles and cannot sustain an excessively rapid respiratory rate. They will tire and subsequently decrease their respiratory rate, indicating development of ventilatory failure. Hypoxemia progresses and respiratory arrest may result if oxygen and/or ventilatory assistance is not provided.

TABLE 3-1 ■ *Normal Vital Signs for Children of Various Age Groups*

AGE GROUP	RESPIRATORY RATE	HEART RATE	SYSTOLIC BLOOD PRESSURE
Newborn	30–50	120–160	50– 70
Infant (1–12 months)	20–30	80–140	70–100
Toddler (1–3 years)	20–30	80–130	80–110
Preschooler (3–5 years)	20–30	80–120	80–110
School Age (6–12 years)	20–30	70–110	80–120
Adolescent (13+ years)	12–20	55–105	100–120

Infants and children under 5 years of age breathe two to three times faster and more shallowly than adults. Both smaller volume and less pressure are needed to ventilate the lungs. Children's tidal volume is proportional to their weight, 5–7 ml/kg, as with adults; therefore, a 12-month-old child weighing 10 kg would have a tidal volume of 70 ml. Only 16–20 cm water pressure (measured by manometer during bag mask ventilation) is usually needed to ventilate a healthy child's lungs. This amount of pressure causes a visible chest rise. Higher pressures will be needed for the initial resuscitation of newborns and for children with diseased lungs (asthma or cystic fibrosis).

Children also have a higher metabolic rate than that of adults, leading to a higher oxygen requirement, 6–8 l/kg/minute in children compared to 3–4 l/kg/minute in an adult. (This is a metabolic oxygen requirement rather than oxygen flow rate used in patient management.) *Hypoxemia*, inadequate oxygen in the arterial blood, develops more rapidly in children when ventilation is compromised.

Heart and Circulation

The child's heart is strong and healthy, unless a congenital heart defect is present. Newborns must make the transition from fetal to pulmonary circulation, usually completed during the first days after birth. Congenital heart defects, such as narrowed valves or abnormal openings between chambers, may result in hypoxemia, respiratory distress, and congestive heart failure in some children.

The normal heart rate varies by age and often increases in response to fear, exercise, *hypoxia* (inadequate oxygen at the cellular level), and hypovolemia. Infants increase their cardiac output principally by increasing their heart rate. As with the respiratory rate, there is a normal heart rate range for children in various age groups (Table 3.1).

- Tachycardia (an excessively high heart rate) is often a response to a demand for more oxygen to the brain. This may result from an increased metabolic rate, such as in a febrile illness, or from hypovolemia due to dehydration or hemorrhage.
- Bradycardia (an excessively low heart rate) is a later response to hypoxia when tachycardia fails to adequately correct tissue hypoxia. Untreated hypoxia and bradycardia leads to respiratory and cardiac arrest. (See page 86.)
- Bradycardia is the initial response to hypoxia in neonates. It is usually a sign of impending cardiac arrest.

The normal range for systolic blood pressure is also related to the age of the child (Table 3.1). Children do not become hypotensive with volume loss as rapidly as do adults. They are able to compensate for a while by increasing vascular resistance by constricting their veins and increasing their heart rate. When these compensating mechanisms are surpassed, as in cases of severe shock, *hypotension will suddenly develop*, usually after a 20 percent or greater volume loss has occurred.

The total circulating blood volume of a child is less than that of an adult; however, children will lose the same amount of blood as an adult from a comparable laceration. Because the child's head is proportionately larger, a greater percentage of the child's total blood volume goes to the head. The child's total blood volume (80–90 ml/kg) is proportional to the body weight (Table 3.2). The newborn, averaging 3.5 kg or 7 lb, thus has approximately 300 ml of blood, slightly more than a cup.

TABLE 3.2 ■ *Total Blood Volume by Age Group and Weight*

Age	Mean Weight		Approximate Blood Volume in ml
	kg	lb	
Newborn	3–5	6–11	240–400
1 Year	10	22	800
3 Years	15	33	1200
5 Years	20	44	1600
8 Years	25	55	2000
10 Years	30	66	2400
15 Years	50	110	4000

Abdomen

Until puberty the child's liver and spleen are proportionately larger and more vascular than an adult's. Because these organs are larger, they are less protected by the rib cage and extend into the abdomen. The ribs are soft and bend easily (compliant), and the child's abdominal muscles are also immature. Both the ribs and abdominal muscles provide these organs with less protection from injury than found in adults. When children experience blunt trauma to the abdomen and lower chest, there is a high index of suspicion for internal injury to these organs.

Extremities

The child's arms and legs grow in length from the growth plates, located near each end of the long bones. Bones start out as cartilage and then harden, or ossify, as minerals are deposited in the cartilage. For this reason, children's bones are softer than those of an adult's; this holds true until puberty. Consequently, children's bones are easily fractured by bending and splintering.

All of the muscle fibers a child develops are present at birth; however, the fibers lengthen and develop throughout childhood as the bones grow.

Nervous System

The child's nervous system develops and matures throughout childhood. The nervous system controls conscious state, communication, motor, coordination, and sensory abilities.

Motor development occurs constantly, proceeding bilaterally in a head-to-toe progression. Motor development occurs in an established pattern, but each child has a personal timetable for achievement of specific functions such as sitting, controlled hand movement, and walking. Coordination is slower to develop and contributes to many falls and injuries.

Sensation is present in all portions of the body at birth. A young infant feels pain but does not have the ability to localize pain and isolate a response to pain to the involved extremity. As nerve connections develop, response to pain becomes much more localized.

Motor and sensory development are most advanced in the cranial nerves at birth because of their life-sustaining function and protective reflexes. These nerves control such functions as blinking, sucking and swallowing, vision, and hearing.

Patient Information

As part of the pediatric assessment, much information about the child's condition will be obtained during scene size-up by observing the environment in which the child is found. Clues in the environment may help the prehospital provider to determine the child's problem. Such clues may include the presence of pill bottles, plants, or household cleaners; position in which the child is found; and a mechanism of injury.

It is equally important to observe the interaction between the child and parent or other care provider. Children generally seek reassurance and comfort from these persons when afraid, ill, or in pain. Passive children who either do not seek or appear to expect such comfort are demonstrating inappropriate behavior. They should be assessed first for an altered level of consciousness. When such a child is alert and conscious, consider the possibility of child abuse or neglect.

The elements of the pediatric history are the same as those collected for adults:

- Reason why EMS was activated.
- Present illness—symptoms and their characteristics according to OPQRST—**O**nset, **P**recipitating events, **Q**uality, **R**adiation, **S**everity, and **T**ime (duration and change in symptoms over time); treatment already attempted; has the child seen a doctor for this problem? (When? What did the doctor say was the problem?)
- Past medical history—significant health problems; any chronic diseases? prematurity, congenital defects, major injuries or surgery, last time the child was at a doctor?
- Medications—those taken for the present illness (including prescription medications and aspirin, Tylenol, or other over-the-counter preparation); when was last dose given? what medications are used routinely for other illnesses?
- Allergies—to foods, medications, plants; type of response.
- Patient's weight—best estimate, or what it was at last visit to doctor.

The SAMPLE mnemonic is one method used by prehospital providers to remember key elements of the patient history.

S = Signs and Symptoms
A = Allergies
M = Medications
P = Pertinent past medical history
L = Last oral intake
E = Events leading up to current problem

If the patient is an infant, some additional information about the health problems of the mother during the pregnancy should be obtained, such as mother's delivery date (premature birth), presence of high blood pressure or vaginal bleeding, and use of any drugs.

For young children, it will be necessary to obtain the history from the parent or care provider. However, once a child is old enough to verbalize, which is about 4 years of age, include the child in the history taking. Ask simple questions the child can understand and answer, such as, "Show me with your finger where it hurts."

Enhancing Cooperation for the Examination

Once the prehospital provider has done a scene size-up for safety and determined that the child has no immediately life-threatening injuries, it is important to gain the child's trust before proceeding with the rest of the examination. The child needs a "transition phase" to become comfortable with the EMT or paramedic and any unfamiliar equipment to be used. *If the child has any life-threatening injuries, intervention begins immediately, without regard for the child's adjustment to the prehospital provider.*

Some units carry teddy bears or dolls to give to small children in their care. If such a toy is not available on your unit, try to use one of the child's favorite toys. A toy like this gives the child something to hold onto for security. It can also be used to obtain a better history from the child, such as pointing out "where it hurts" (Figure 3.6).

To reassure the nonacutely ill child, project a calm and friendly manner. Whenever possible, speak to the child at the child's eye level. Include the child in the conversation with the parent. Ask questions such as "What happened?" "How do you feel?" "Can you point with one finger to where it hurts?" Avoid asking questions with yes or no answers when possible. When speaking to the child, use age-appropriate language and a quiet tone of voice.

Certain words may cause more anxiety in a child and should be avoided, if possible, even in discussions with your partner. *Cut* implies pain; *laceration* will not be understood by young children and may cause less anxiety to the child when discussing care with your partner.

FIGURE 3.6 During the patient interview, speak to the child in a calm voice at the child's eye level. Provide a security toy, which can be used to improve communication with the child.

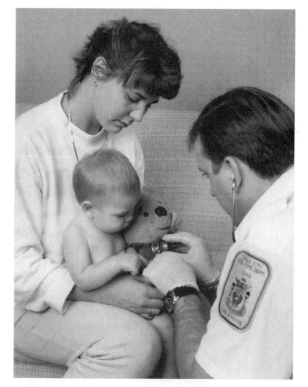

Chapter 3: General Pediatric Assessment

Take, as in "take a blood pressure," implies removal of something. Alternate wording to explain this procedure to the child could be "measure how hard your heart is working." *Bleeding* may cause children to think that all their blood will leak out.

Smile at the child frequently and project confidence. Look at your patient periodically, rather than staring at him or her. Children may perceive staring as threatening and become more afraid. Make sure young patients have their security toys or provide a toy to distract them. Whenever possible, keep the child with the parent for the examination.

Be honest when explaining, in simple terms, what you are going to do. If a procedure will hurt, explain this just prior to doing it, and say it will be over soon. However, do not inform the child about expected pain too soon, as the fear of pain increases with the length of the wait. Expect children to be distressed about a painful procedure, but most will cope better if informed. The child also benefits by learning to trust your honestly for the remainder of your care.

To gain the child's cooperation for the use of instruments during the examination, let the child handle or play with the equipment (Figure 3.7). Demonstrate how the equipment works on the parent, the EMT, or the child's toy. Try to explain the equipment in nonthreatening terms:

- A penlight is a candle that can be blown out.
- A stethoscope is a telephone.
- A blood pressure cuff is a balloon, and the dial is a clock.

Examine the child seated on the parent's lap, facing you (Figure 3.8). If an infant or toddler becomes distressed, place him or her over the parent's shoulder, facing away from you. Auscultation of the chest can be done successfully through the back because the chest wall is thin in children. You can then walk around the parent's back to look at the infant's face for other assessment parameters. When touching the child, begin at the feet, proceeding to the head. The child may develop more trust if less-threatening anatomy is examined first. Make sure your motions are slow and deliberate.

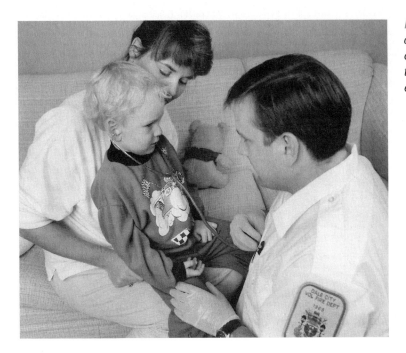

FIGURE 3.7 To enhance cooperation during the examination, permit the child who is not critically ill or injured to become familiar with the examining equipment.

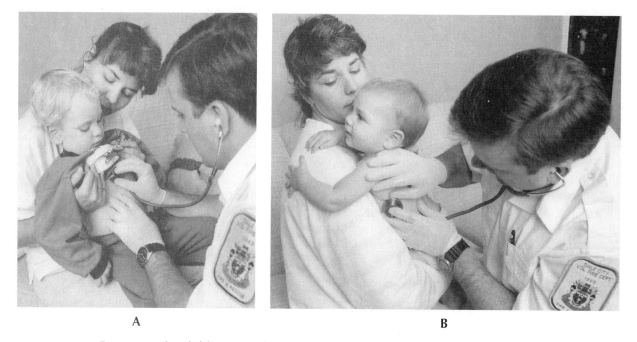

A   B

FIGURE 3.8   Encourage the child's sense of security during the examination by keeping the child with the parent. (A) Examine the toddler on the parent's lap. (B) Examine the infant who is held across the parent's shoulder.

A number of factors will contribute to your success in completing all aspects of the examination. Examination of the child will be more difficult in any of the following situations:

- If the child has had a bad prior experience with a health care provider;
- If the child has been told to stay away from or not talk to strangers;
- If the child is not old enough to understand the reasons for what you are doing;
- If a parent is not present to reassure the child;
- If the child has been taught that certain parts of his or her body should not be touched by a stranger.

If the child becomes uncooperative in spite of your best efforts to reduce the child's anxiety, you should complete what you can of the assessment and transport. It is fruitless to waste more time. Remember to take advantage of assessment opportunities, even if the child is uncooperative. Observation of the crying child will provide a lot of information:

- Quality of the cry
- An open mouth to evaluate color and hydration
- A deep breath as the child inspires to evaluate breath sounds
- Symmetry of facial expression
- Presence or absence of tears.

Physical Examination and Interpretation of Findings

Inspection, auscultation, and palpation are the examination techniques most frequently used during the initial assessment and detailed physical exam. This section describes the procedures for patient assessment and interpretation of findings. The sequence of the assessment used should be the same taught in all prehospital training programs. See Chapter 9, "Trauma," for the correct approach.

In every case, you will perform your initial assessment to detect the presence of any life-threatening problem.

- Listening to the child's cry, voice, and breathing provides information about the status of the airway and ventilation.
- Observing the child's skin color and assessing capillary refill provides information about circulation, if not in a cold environment.
- Observing the child's interest (orientation or mental status) during the assessment provides clues about the level of responsiveness.

Weight of the Child

If the parent or caretaker is unable to provide you with an estimate of the child's weight, it will be necessary to make your own estimate using a length-based resuscitation tape, such as the Broselow. Parents generally know their child's weight in pounds, but drug dosages are calculated by weight in kilograms. The conversion factor is 2.2 lb = 1 kg, or refer to Table 3.2. Remember to carry a conversion chart into the field. While children come in various weights for their age, one formula to estimate the child's weight in kilograms is as follows:

$8 + (2 \times$ the child's age)

A 5-year-old child would then weigh approximately 18 kg.

$8 + (2 \times 5) = 18$ kg

Skin Condition

The color of a child's skin provides clues about tissue perfusion. To best assess the generalized color in all children, observe the palms of the hands and the mucous membranes in the mouth.

- Pallor may indicate poor tissue perfusion.
- Localized flushing or redness may indicate inflammation.
- A mottled appearance is associated with hypoxia or hypothermia.
- Cyanosis is most often associated with a congenital heart defect, but may be present in cases of severe hypoxemia associated with respiratory distress.
- During their transition to extrauterine life, newborns often have cyanotic feet and hands while the rest of the body is pink (acrocyanosis).
- Jaundice, yellowing of the sclerae of the eyes and skin, is associated with hepatitis and a congenital liver defect.

Look for signs of tissue injury, such as bruises, burns, abrasions, lacerations, bleeding, and inflammation. Note their distribution and any special characteristics. The age of a bruise can be estimated by its color (Table 3.3).

The resilience of the skin (turgor) and dryness of the mucous membranes in the mouth provide clues about the hydration status of the child. Pinch some skin between your finger and thumb and let it go. The skin should immediately return to its previous contour (Figure 3.9). Any delay in this return, or tenting, indicates poor skin turgor and moderate to severe dehydration. In cases of moderate dehydration it will take 2 to 4 seconds for tented skin to return to its natural shape. In cases of severe

TABLE 3.3 ■ *Assessing the Age of Bruises*

COLOR	APPROXIMATE AGE OF BRUISE
Reddish blue	Up to 48 hours
Brownish blue	2 to 3 days
Brownish green	4 to 7 days
Greenish yellow	7 to 10 days
Yellow brown	More than 8 days
Normal Skin Color	2 to 4 weeks

Source: Adapted from Wilson, E.F. (1977): "Estimating the age of cutaneous contusions in child abuse," *Pediatrics,* 60: 750.

dehydration it will take more than 4 seconds. Dry or parched mucous membranes also indicate dehydration.

Moist skin may be related to perspiration associated with exercise, high external temperatures, and fever. The child with an uncorrected congenital heart defect may have profuse sweating with minimal activity, such as feeding.

Skin temperature can be assessed by placing the back of your hand against the child's forehead and extremities. Temperature strips, if available, can be used to get a more specific temperature reading. Cool, pale extremities are associated with hypoperfusion (shock), hypothermia, and a cold environment. Flushed, warm skin is associated with a fever.

Mental Status

Level of responsiveness is initially assessed by determining how alert the child is. Infants and young children who are not verbal must be observed for activity and interest in what is happening. The infant and young child who is irritable and cannot be consoled by the parent has an altered level

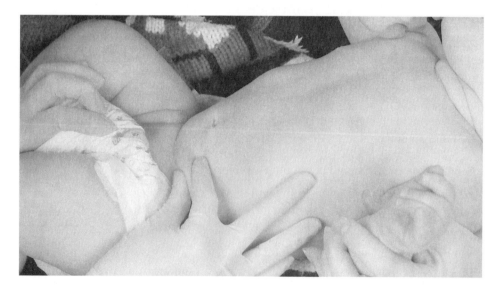

FIGURE 3.9 *Testing for skin turgor. Pinch some skin between your finger and thumb and release it. Watch to see if the skin immediately returns as expected to its previous contour.*

of responsiveness. Parents are often able to tell you if the child is not as alert as usual.

The AVPU mnemonic is useful in the initial assessment of mental status.

Alert—Children are curious and usually vigilant when approached by a stranger.

Responsive to **V**erbal stimuli—The child is uninterested in events or dozing (lethargic), but responds by turning the head or stopping activity in response to sound.

Responsive to **P**ainful stimuli—The child is hard to arouse (stuporous), but moans or moves when pinched.

Unresponsive—The child does not respond to any stimuli.

Respiratory Assessment

A crying or talking child has a patent airway, at least at that time. Listen to the quality of the child's speech to gain other clues about the child's problems.

- Hoarseness may be caused by a foreign body or inflammation associated with an upper airway disease.
- Moaning is associated with shock and a decreasing level of consciousness.
- A high-pitched cry is associated with increased intracranial pressure.

Observe the child's face for nasal flaring, which is the body's attempt to expand the size of the airway to move more air. Also observe the child's facial expression. *Children who are anxious and focused on breathing, rather than demonstrating interest in what is happening around them, are in acute respiratory distress* (Figure 3.10). Listen for other sounds that can be heard without a stethoscope.

- Stridor is a hoarse voice or cry and a seal-like barking cough that is heard on inspiration and expiration. It is associated with a foreign body and inflammation in the glottic area of the trachea.
- Wheezing is the passage of expired air over mucous secretions that have collected in the bronchi during bronchospasm.
- Whistling or noisy breathing may be heard on inspiration and expiration and may be associated with a partial airway obstruction.
- Grunting is a sound in which an infant attempts to build back pressure during expiration to keep the alveoli open. It indicates severe respiratory distress in newborns.
- Bubbling or gurgling may indicate an open chest wound.

Observe the movement of the chest with respirations. There should be bilateral chest rise with each breath, even if it is subtle. Note the presence of any retractions and their location (intercostal, suprasternal, and sternal). These indicate increased effort with breathing. There should be a synchronized rise of the chest and abdomen with each breath. See-saw respirations, in which the child's chest falls (sternal retraction) as the abdomen rises and vice versa, indicate severe respiratory distress.

Count the respiratory rate by observing the abdomen rise. Make this assessment prior to touching the child to obtain the most accurate rate. Often touching the child will increase the child's anxiety and lead to an acceleration in the respiratory rate.

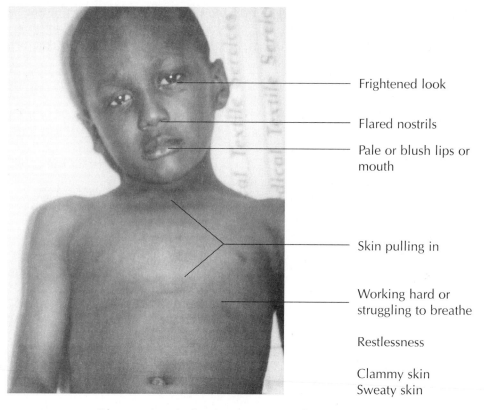

Frightened look

Flared nostrils

Pale or blush lips or mouth

Skin pulling in

Working hard or struggling to breathe

Restlessness

Clammy skin
Sweaty skin

FIGURE 3.10   Observe signs indicating respiratory distress.

Listen to breath sounds with the stethoscope. A pediatric stethoscope is not necessary; the bell of an adult stethoscope pressed firmly to the skin so the skin fills the bell will create a pediatric diaphragm. Because the chest wall is so thin in children, breath sounds are disseminated from one side of the chest to the other. Place the diaphragm of the stethoscope in the axillae along the midaxillary line and just under the clavicles in the midclavicular line (Figure 3.11). Listening in these locations provides the best chance to hear local breath sounds rather than the sounds transmitted from the other lung. If a child is crying, be patient and listen for the breath sounds at the end of each cry when the child inspires. The breath sounds should be present bilaterally.

Circulatory Assessment

Capillary refill is a good indicator of circulatory perfusion in children and one of the best indicators of early hypoperfusion (shock). Press on the child's nailbed for a couple of seconds and release. A pink return to the blanched tissue should occur within 2 seconds, or the time it takes to say "capillary refill." Alternate sites for capillary refill assessment are the forehead, chin, sternum, or gums or the mouth (Figure 3.12). These alternate sites should be used in any child in a cold environment or suspected of hypoperfusion or hypothermia, when vasoconstriction to the extremities is present.

Observe for any lacerations or bleeding. Assess the amount of blood loss in relation to the child's total blood volume, generally estimated to be 80 ml/kg (Table 3.2, page 32).

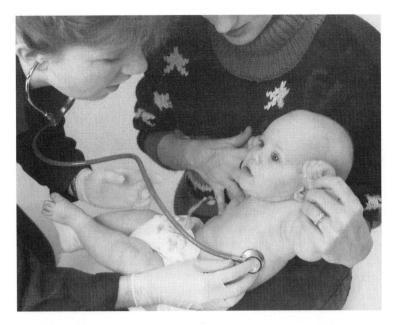

FIGURE 3.11 Assess breath sounds by placing the stethoscope along the midaxillary line as demonstrated here and just under the clavicles in the mid-clavicular line.

Count the child's heart rate. For infants, palpate either the brachial or femoral pulse, or auscultate the apical pulse. The infant's neck is so short that it is difficult to palpate the carotid pulse. Older children can have their carotid pulse palpated. Because the chest wall is so thin, it is also possible to auscultate the heart through the back when the child is held over the parent's shoulder.

The quality of distal pulses should be assessed, but these sites are the least accurate to use when determining the heart rate of a child under 4 years of age. Children readily vasoconstrict blood vessels in their extremities, and distal pulses become hard to palpate. If the brachial and femoral pulses are weak in a child, this is an indicator of severe shock.

Children's heart rates will vary by age and with respirations. Heart rate increases on inspiration and decreases on expiration. The child's myocardium is generally strong and dysrhythmias are uncommon. Bradycardia and asystole are the two most common dysrhythmias. Make sure to note any rate irregularities.

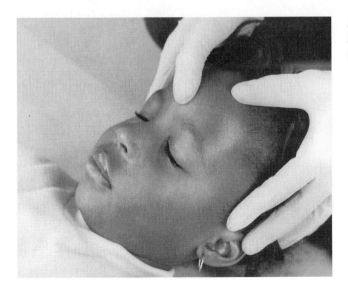

FIGURE 3.12 Assessment of capillary refill time by pressing the skin over a bony prominence (forehead, sternum, chin) or over a nailbed.

When taking a child's blood pressure, the cuff or bladder size is the most important variable in obtaining an accurate reading. Blood pressure cuffs come in numerous sizes; thus it is necessary to determine the one most appropriate for the child you are assessing:

- The bladder should not overlap when wrapped around the extremity, but should cover at least two-thirds of the circumference.
- The width of the cuff should be about two-thirds of the length of the long bone used (upper arm, lower arm, thigh).

If the cuff you have does not fit one extremity in the child, such as the upper arm, see if it can be used on the thigh.

It may be difficult to get an accurate blood pressure reading when the child does not cooperate, as often occurs in children under 3 years of age. Emotional upset, fear, and anxiety will all increase the systolic reading. In some cases it will be difficult to auscultate the blood pressure because of extrinsic noise, unless an ultrasound doppler is available. The systolic reading may then be estimated by a palpation. While there are ranges of blood pressure by age group, a formula to estimate the appropriate blood pressure in a child over 1 year of age is:

$$80 + (2 \times \text{the child's age [years]}) = \text{systolic BP}$$

The diastolic reading should be approximately two-thirds of the systolic reading.

If you are unable to obtain an accurate blood pressure reading, especially in children under 3 years of age, assess the perfusion status of the child, using the following indicators:

- heart rate
- capillary refill, at either a distal or central location
- extremity warmth
- mental status.

Abdomen

The contour of the abdomen should be observed when the child is supine. It is usually rounded in children. A sunken abdomen in a newborn should alert you to the possibility of a hiatal hernia, a life-threatening congenital defect.

Observe for any discolorations on the abdomen such as bruises or bluish discoloration around the umbilicus (Cullen's sign) or along the flanks. These signs may indicate intra-abdominal bleeding.

Lightly palpate the abdomen, noting any expression of pain on the child's face or guarding as you palpate (Figure 3.13). Do not rely on young children to tell you when it hurts. They will often say it hurts when they feel you touching or tickling them.

Extremities

Observe the alignment of the arms and legs, noting any deformity that might indicate a fracture. The alignment should by symmetric, when comparing extremities on each side. Carefully inspect for any open wounds in the area of a suspected fracture, which would indicate an open fracture.

Palpate each extremity, noting any deformity or pain. Palpate the distal pulse; check capillary refill time and the presence of sensation whenever a fracture is suspected prior to and immediately after any manipulation of the extremity. Compare your findings with those on the opposite extremity.

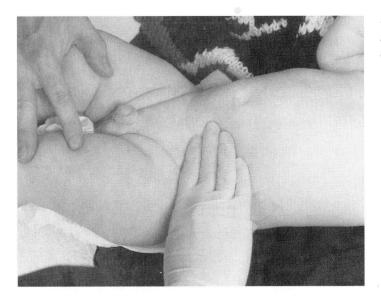

Neurologic Assessment

Cranial nerves are important to evaluate in the child, especially in the case of head injury, because they originate in the brain. They control the movement and sensation of the head and neck, and special senses such as vision, hearing, smell, and taste.

- Observe the child's face for symmetry of facial features when the child smiles or cries.
- Observe eye movement by having the child look at a penlight or toy as you move it slowly from one side of the child's face to the other. Make sure the child's head does not move.
- Use the penlight to check pupils for size and reaction to light.
- A response to questions or turning the head to noise indicates the presence of hearing.
- Infants should be able to suck and swallow from a bottle in a coordinated way without choking. However, do not feed a head-injured infant to assess this cranial nerve.

The Glasgow Coma Scale can be used to quantify the level of consciousness. It must be slightly modified for use with infants. The two categories that have different criteria for scoring are *verbal response* and *motor response*. (See Table 3.4 for the recommended modification for infants.)

The integrity of the child's motor function can be tested by observing the voluntary, purposeful movement of the extremities. Infants under 4 months of age can have motor function tested by the palmar grasp reflex. Place your finger into the palm of the infant's hands (Figure 3.14). There should be an immediate grasp around your finger, equal in strength on each side. Offer a toy to the toddler and watch him or her take it. Test strength by seeing how tightly the child holds on to the toy. The same information can be obtained by watching the child cling to the parent or attempt to get away from you. The child over 3 years of age will often follow directions and squeeze your finger or push your hand away if you approach this like a game.

Sensation can be tested by lightly stroking each arm and leg with your finger. This often stimulates a ticklish response from which the child attempts to withdraw. There should be equal movement bilaterally.

TABLE 3.4 ■ *Glasgow Coma Scale Modifications for Infants*

CATEGORY	RESPONSE	SCORE
Verbal	Happy, coos, babbles, or cries spontaneously	5
	Irritable crying, but consolable	4
	Cries to pain, weak cry	3
	Moans to pain	2
	None	1
Motor	Spontaneous movement	6
	Withdraws to touch	5
	Withdraws to pain	4
	Abnormal flexion	3
	Abnormal extension	2
	None	1
Eye Opening (same as adult)	Spontaneous	4
	To speech	3
	To pain	2
	None	1

Source: Adapted from James, H.E. (1986): "Neurologic evaluation and support in the child with acute brain insult," *Pediatric Annals,* 15(1): 17.

Signs Associated with Common Pediatric Emergencies

Once you have completed your examination of the child, it is then necessary to put signs together to determine what is wrong with the young patient and the severity of the problem (Table 3.5). Some signs fall together in a classic pattern to assist you in making your assessment (Table 3.6).

FIGURE 3.14 Test motor function in the young infant with the palmar grasp reflex. Place your finger into the palm of the infant's hands, which should be followed by an immediate grasp around your finger.

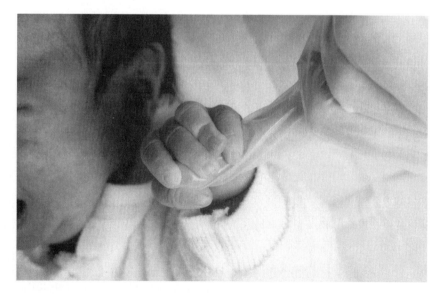

TABLE 3.5 ■ *Signs Indicating Severity of Illness in Children*

Physical Sign	Normal	Moderately Ill	Seriously Ill
Color	Pink	Pale	Mottled, cyanotic
Hydration	Moist mucous membranes, good skin turgor, flat fontanelles, light-colored urine	Sticky mucous membranes, slightly doughy skin turgor, slightly sunken fontanelle, dark-colored urine	Dry mucous membranes, tenting skin turgor, depressed fontanelle, sunken eyes, no urine
Response to Stimulation	Arouses easily, then stays awake and alert	Arouses to repeated gentle stimulation, may fall back to sleep quickly when stimulus stops	Arouses only with aggressive or irritating stimulation, or does not arouse at all
Behavior	Unchanged	Fussy, but can be comforted	Irritable and inconsolable if awake
Cry	Unchanged	Whimpers, sobs, or whines	High-pitched and screeching, or weak and moaning

Source: Henderson, D.P., and Brownstein, D., eds. *Pediatric Emergency Nursing Manual.* New York: Springer Publishing Company, 1994. Used with permission.

TABLE 3.6 ■ *Classic Patterns of Signs Indicating Various Physiologic Problems*

Pain
Shallow breathing
Irritable crying
Splinting (Avoiding movement)
Facial expression change when
    touched or moved
Resists movement
Rigid posturing

Respiratory Distress
Nasal flaring
Mottled, dusky skin color
Tachypnea, shallow breathing
Altered level of consciousness
Sounds—stridor, hoarseness, muffled voice, wheezing
Tripod positioning
Retractions
Asymmetric chest movement
"See-saw" respirations

Early Shock
Tachycardia > 130/minute
Capillary refill > 2 seconds
Pale, cool skin
Altered level of consciousness
Normal systolic blood pressure

Late Shock
Tachycardia > 130/minute
Capillary refill > 3–4 seconds
Pallor, cold extremities
Altered level of consciousness
Systolic BP < 80 mmHg (except infants whose systolic
    BP is often normally lower)

Moderate Dehydration
Sunken fontanelle
Pallor
Doughy skin texture
Dry mucous membranes

Severe Dehydration
Sunken fontanelle
Signs of shock
Parched mucous membranes
No tears
Sunken eyeballs

Altered Level of Consciousness
Combative
Decreased responsiveness
Lethargy
Weak cry, moaning
Personality change

Increased Intracranial Pressure
Bulging fontanelle
Altered level of consciousness
High-pitched cry
Change in vital signs
Irritable cry, unable to distract or console child

Assessment References

Chameides, L., and Hazinski, M.F., eds., *Textbook of Pediatric Advanced Life Support*, 2nd ed. Dallas: American Heart Association, 1994.

Dierking, B.H., and Ramenofsky, M.L., "Obtaining a pediatric medical history: A prehospital approach to history-taking," *JEMS*, 14, no. 3 (March 1988), pp. 61–63.

Henderson, D.P., and Brownstein, D., eds., *Pediatric Emergency Nursing Manual.* New York: Springer Publishing Company, 1994.

James, H.E., "Neurologic evaluation and support in the child with acute brain insult," *Pediatric Annals*, 15, no. 1 (January 1986), p. 17.

Mellick, L.B., and Guy, J.R., "Approaching the infant and child in the prehospital arena," *JEMS*, 18, no. 3 (March 1992), pp. 126–136.

Murphy, P.M., "Pint-size patients: Gaining confidence in assessing peds," *JEMS*, 21, no. 3 (March 1996), pp. 103–114.

Seidel, H.M., Ball, J.B., et al., *Mosby's Guide to Physical Examination*, 3rd ed. St. Louis: Mosby Year Book, Inc., 1995.

Equipment and Procedures for Management of ABCs

OBJECTIVES

When you have completed this chapter you should be able to

▶ Describe the anatomic and physiologic considerations in the management of the child's airway.
▶ Describe effective airway management with basic life-support maneuvers.
▶ Identify techniques for packaging an injured child that protect the airway, breathing, and cervical spine.
▶ Describe advanced airway and respiratory management of the child to include the following:
  • Endotracheal intubation
  • Cricothyrotomy
  • Pleural decompression
▶ Describe the procedures to obtain a fluid route in the pediatric patient to include the following:
  • Peripheral lines
  • Umbilical vein cannulation
  • Intraosseous infusion
▶ List the steps in the procedure for defibrillation and cardioversion of the pediatric patient.

The purpose of the respiratory system is to deliver oxygen to the lungs and remove carbon dioxide. It maintains a delicate balance within the body, making adjustments on a continuous basis. The ability of the respiratory system to regulate change assures a constant and precise exchange of gases. The airway must be open for gas exchange to occur.

Therefore, it is essential for all emergency providers to master the skill of airway management. This is accomplished by having a thorough understanding of the anatomy and physiology of the airway and respiratory system, as well as those management techniques and adjuncts used in the assessment and treatment.

Anatomy and Physiology

The chapter on general pediatric assessment provides a thorough review of the pediatric respiratory system as well as all other body systems. It is suggested that a review of that chapter be completed prior to this section.

There are several anatomical features that make the pediatric airway unique, requiring familiarity to manage the child's airway (Figure 3.3). They are as follows:

- Nasal openings are smaller.
- The tongue is large in proportion to the oral cavity.
- The trachea is short and narrow.
- The larynx is higher and more anterior.
- The nose and face are flat.
- The secretions are copious.
- The tracheal cartilage is more elastic.
- The occiput is large.

With these unique features of the pediatric airway committed to memory, you can next concentrate on management with the appropriate adjunct and technique.

Plan of Action for Airway Control

The goal of airway management is to achieve adequate oxygenation. This can be accomplished with a variety of maneuvers and equipment, from very simple to very complex. In planning airway management, a solid plan of action needs to be established, which includes an assessment of the child's current airway status and the possible future needs of this patient. A seven-step plan of action from simple to complex should be implemented for every child that presents with respiratory distress or an uncontrolled airway.

1. Reposition the airway
2. Suction
3. Bag-mask ventilation
4. Oral airway
5. Nasal airway for child over 8 years of age
6. Endotracheal intubation
7. Cricothyrotomy or Surgical Airway

After assuring the scene is safe and noting any mechanism of injury, manually opening the airway is the first step. Because of the child's large

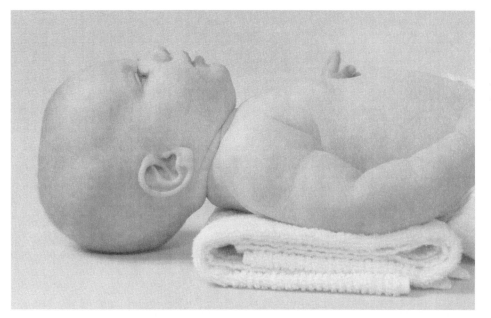

head, there is a tendency for the trachea to become flexed when the child is supine. A small pillow or towel placed underneath the shoulders raises the shoulders and straightens the neck, so the child is in neutral alignment, or "sniffing" position (the slight extension of the neck associated with sniffing a flower) (Figure 4.1).

Extreme vigilance is necessary to maintain an open airway in the pediatric patient, especially since the tongue is the most common airway obstruction in infants and children. The preferred method to reposition and open the airway is the head-tilt, chin-lift. If a cervical spine injury is suspected, the preferred method is the jaw thrust with in-line stabilization. Because the tongue follows the mandible, both of these maneuvers pull the tongue forward, out of the posterior oral pharynx, opening the airway. Avoid putting pressure on the soft tissues below the mandible that may defeat any measures to open the airway (Figure 4.2). If the airway is still not patent after these maneuvers, consider a partial or complete foreign body obstruction and treat accordingly.

Suctioning is the next step if the airway is still uncontrolled. If the patient continues with inadequate air exchange, then assist the patient with bag-mask ventilation with 100% oxygen. When the child is unconscious without a gag-reflex, an oral or nasal airway may be inserted. Continued airway instability requires endotracheal intubation or, as a last resort, cricothyrotomy, or surgical airway.

This plan of action in anticipating the potential airway management needs of the patient works well by following the simple to the more complex management options. It is important to proceed from the most simple airway maneuver on up because of the potential complications associated with more complex maneuvers.

Airway Adjuncts

As a rescuer you are provided with an arsenal of equipment to manage the airway. By using this equipment, along with the knowledge you already possess and the information provided in this text, you will be optimally prepared to manage the pediatric airway.

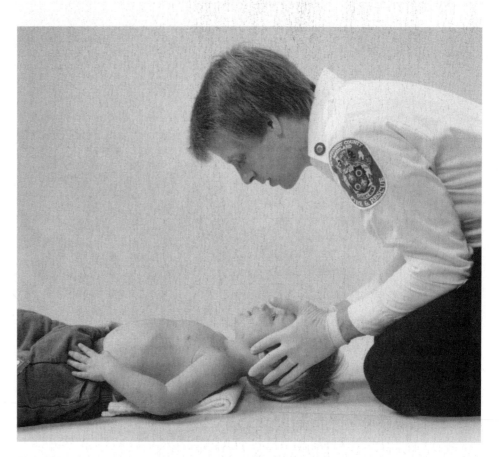

FIGURE 4.2   *Jaw-thrust maneuver. Note the simultaneous in-line stabilization of the C-spine.*

Oxygen

Normal atmospheric concentration of oxygen is 21%. Prehospital providers have the ability to increase the concentration anywhere from 24% to 100%, depending on the selection of adjuncts. To start, there must be an adequate supply of oxygen. Other highly desirable characteristics are humidified or heated oxygen.

- Humidified oxygen prevents the mucous membranes of the airway from drying and becoming thick with secretions.
- Heated oxygen is particularly beneficial in cold climates and management of children with hypothermia. When cold oxygen is blown on their faces in the distribution of the trigeminal nerve, newborns and young infants also have the diving reflex triggered, causing apnea and bradycardia.

Unfortunately, warmed or humidified oxygen is often unavailable in the prehospital setting. This should not delay or preclude the rescuer from administering oxygen.

Oxygen Delivery Devices

The nasal cannula is a plastic tube with two plastic prongs that can be inserted into the anterior portion of the nares. With a flow rate of 2–6 l/min, a concentration of 24–50% is achieved. Increasing the flow rate will not increase the concentration, but will only lead to increased irritation of

Chapter 4: Equipment and Procedures for Management of ABCs

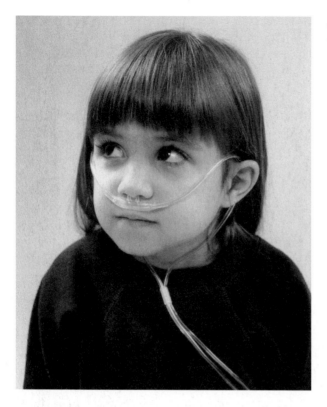

FIGURE 4.3   Delivery of oxygen via nasal cannula in the school-age child.

the nose and throat. Position the nasal cannula in the pediatric patient, making sure the prongs do not fit in the nostril too tightly. If blanching of the nostril is constant, then the prong is too large and should be removed. An alternate position might be to rest the prongs on the ridge of the lip, pointed toward the nostril (Figure 4.3). The nasal cannula should be used in the older child or adolescent and is not adaptive to the younger child.

The simple face mask (Figure 4.4A) is a plastic mask designed to fit over the nose and mouth of the patient. The mask has vents on the side

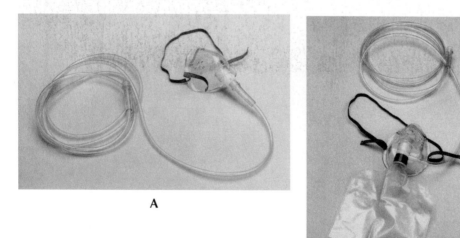

A

B

FIGURE 4.4   (A) Simple face mask. (B) Nonrebreather mask.

that allow for air to be exhaled. At a flow rate of 6–10 l/min, the concentration will vary from 30–60%. This variation is dependent on the patient's respiratory rate and depth of respiration. The more external air entering the mask, the lower the concentration. As a rule, this type of mask should have a minimum liter flow of 6 l/min to achieve higher levels of oxygen concentration.

The nonrebreather mask is equipped with a reservoir bag and a one-way valve that allows inspiration of oxygen and expiration of gases. With a flow rate of 10–15 l/min, this mask will deliver 90–100% oxygen when fitted properly (Figure 4.4B).

Special Considerations

Placing one of these adjuncts on a pediatric patient can be trying in itself. Some points to remember include the following:

- Always explain what you are doing to the patient. Children are afraid of everything involved in this situation. An explanation, and possibly a demonstration, can go a long way to comfort the young patient. Use the parents to demonstrate placement of the mask.
- Some children will not tolerate a mask because they feel it is suffocating them. In this case, the mask can be held in front of the child by the parent, or perhaps even the child if he or she is able to do so.
- If the child still resists, try a nasal cannula. Some oxygen is better than no oxygen.
- In delivering oxygen to an infant, care should be taken not to blow the oxygen directly onto the face. The infant has an immature nervous system, and stimulation of the nerves around the mouth and nose with cold oxygen could trigger a slowing of the respiratory and heart rates. The recommended method of delivering oxygen is the blow-by method. This can be done by placing the oxygen tubing through the bottom of a paper cup, and holding the cup to one side of the infant's face, about 4 to 6 inches away (see Figure 4.5).

FIGURE 4.5 Delivery of oxygen, using blow-by method.

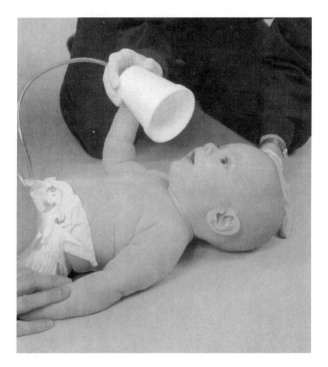

Chapter 4: Equipment and Procedures for Management of ABCs

Oral and Nasal Airways

The oropharyngeal airway is a curved plastic tube that can be inserted into the mouth to hold the tongue off the back of the throat. It should be used only in the unconscious patient without a gag reflex. Pediatric sizes range from 000–4.

Measurement of the oral airway is the most important step in the process. An oral airway that is too long will rest against the epiglottis, obstructing the airway completely. An oral airway that is too short will push the tongue back into the posterior pharynx, resulting in a completely obstructed airway. The proper method of measurement and insertion is as follows:

- To select the proper-size oral airway, place it near the face between the ear and mouth. Choose the oral airway that most closely fits in the space from the angle of the jaw to the crease of the mouth (Figure 4.6A).
- Using a tongue depressor, press down the tongue and insert the airway in the position of function (Figure 4.6B, C). There is potential for damage to the soft tissues of the mouth if the oral airway is inserted upside down and rotated.
- Assess for good air exchange.

The nasopharyngeal airway is a soft rubber tube that is inserted through the nose into the posterior pharynx. This allows air to pass from

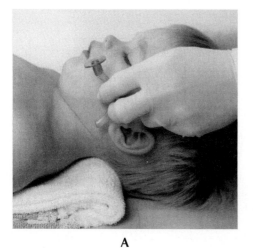

A

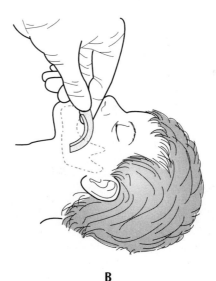

B

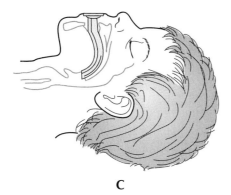

C

FIGURE 4.6 (A) Selecting correct size of oral airway: Length should equal distance from crease of mouth to angle of jaw. (B) Insertion of oral airway in anatomically correct position, using a tongue blade. (C) Proper placement of the airway.

the nose to the lung. The airway is available in sizes 12 to 36 French. A 12 French is about the size of a 3 mm endotracheal tube and should fit a full-term infant. The nasopharyngeal airway should be inserted as follows:

- Select the appropriately sized airway. The length should fit the space from the tip of the nose to the tragus of the ear. The size of the airway can be determined by the size of the child's little finger or external naris opening (Figure 4.7A, B).
- Lubricate the airway with a water-based lubricant.
- Insert the airway gently into the nostril in the position of function and slide it along the floor of the nasopharynx (Figure 4.7C).
- If resistance is felt, don't force the airway. This may lacerate the tissues, resulting in hemorrhage that will further complicate airway management.
- The diameter of the airway is too large if it causes blanching at the naris. If this occurs, remove the airway and replace it with a smaller size.

Suction

Achieving adequate air exchange often requires suctioning secretions from the airway. Suctioning can be provided by manual or electrical sources. The bulb syringe and mechanical units each have merit for suctioning the narrow, fragile airways of the infant.

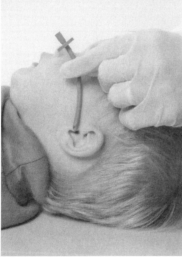

A

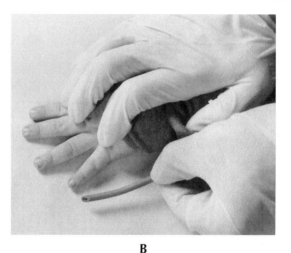

B

FIGURE 4.7 *(A) Selecting the correct size of the nasopharyngeal airway length should equal the distance from the nasal opening to the tragus of the ear. (B) Circumference of the nasopharyngeal airway should equal the size of the child's little finger. (C) Proper placement of the nasopharyngeal airway.*

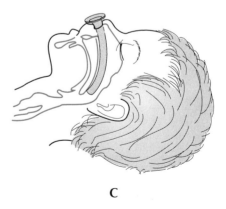

C

Bulb-Syringe Technique

- Place the bulb syringe in your hand and squeeze out the air.
- Place the nipple of the bulb into either the nostril or the mouth. Secure a form-fitting seal and release.
- Remove the syringe and expel the contents.
- Repeat the procedure as needed (Figure 4.8).

Mechanical Suction

- Select the appropriate suction device. A flexible catheter should range in diameter size from 10 to 16 French. A hard catheter (tonsil tip) is very effective to clear obstructions in the mouth of infants (Figure 4.9).
- Flexible catheters can be placed either in the nose or the mouth, but hard catheters should be used only in the mouth.
- Apply suction for no more than 5 seconds, withdrawing the catheter in a circular motion. Suctioning the infant or child for longer time periods may stimulate a vagal response, thus slowing the heart and respiratory rates.
- Oxygenate between each suctioning attempt and closely monitor the vital signs.

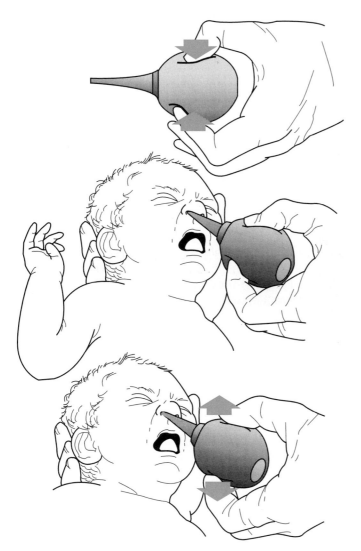

FIGURE 4.8   Bulb-syringe suctioning of infant. Squeeze the bulb prior to placing the nipple to the infant's nose.

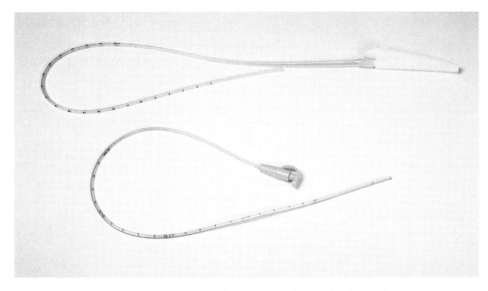

FIGURE 4.9   Suctioning devices: Soft suction catheter, feeding tube.

Assisting Ventilation

Bag-Mask Ventilation

The objective in bag-mask ventilation is to augment respirations or provide complete assistance in respiratory failure. The inspired oxygen concentration should be as close to 100% as possible. The bag-valve mask is the preferred ventilatory equipment for infants and children. You can manage the airway more effectively by assessing the rise and fall of the chest and lung compliance, securing a constant mask seal, and providing vigilant supervision of the airway. The importance of proper bag-valve-mask use cannot be over emphasized. You must be familiar with parts of the bag-valve mask and assemble and select an appropriate-sized mask (Figure 4.10).

- Make sure the bag has a constant source of 100% oxygen. An oxygen reservoir, or a pressure demand valve should be hooked into the bag to ensure refilling of oxygen (Figure 4.10 A,B).
- Select a clear mask. This will enable you to visualize vomitus, blood, or other secretions that may cause airway obstruction.
- Select the appropriate-sized mask. The mask should fit over the bridge of the nose to the cleft of the chin (Figure 4.11).
- Position the head in neutral alignment or sniffing position. It may be helpful to place a folded towel under the child's shoulders to compensate for the child's large occiput and to maintain neutral alignment of the airway and cervical spine. This extra padding is usually necessary until around the age of 8 years.
- Securing the mask to the face with a tight seal is essential for ventilation. To assure a tight seal with the mask:
  1. Wrap the index finger and thumb, in the shape of a "C," around the mask where it connects with the bag.
  2. Place the middle, ring, and little fingers along the lower jaw and hook them underneath the bony prominence of the mandible.

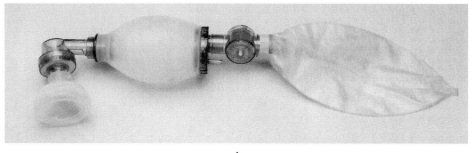

A

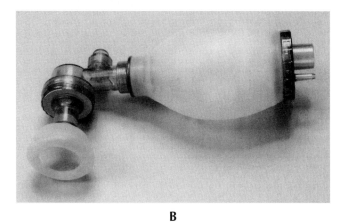

B

FIGURE 4.10
Self-inflating bag.
(A) with an oxygen
reservoir. (B) Without
an oxygen reservoir.

Infants and small children only require that the middle finger be used in hooking the jaw. The ring finger and little finger should be folded out of the way (Figure 4.12).

■ Do not press on the soft tissue underneath the chin. This will cause the tongue to obstruct the airway.

■ Gently pull the patient's face up to the mask while maintaining a neutral or sniffing position.

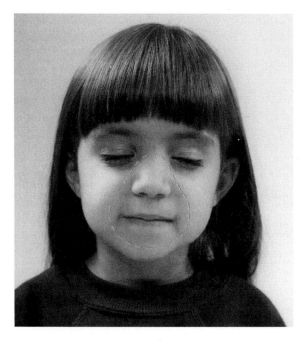

FIGURE 4.11   Choose a
proper-fitting mask that covers
the mouth and nose and seals
around the facial features.

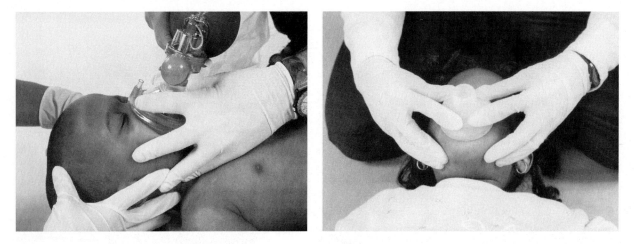

FIGURE 4.12 *Proper hand and finger placement to hold a face mask in position for ventilation. (A) One-handed technique with a second person stabilizing the cervical spine, (B) Two-handed technique; a second person is needed to ventilate.*

- Squeeze the bag and ventilate the patient, assessing the quality of respiration and making adjustments as needed.
- If an adequate seal is not maintained, you may need to place both hands on the mask to assure a tight seal.

Ventilate the infant or child with only enough pressure to make the chest rise at a rate equivalent to the child's expected respiratory rate, or higher if the patient's condition warrants it. Use even, gentle pressure to ventilate; only enough to see chest rise. Provide ventilation with a 1:2 inspiration: expiration ratio. This provides an optimal time for oxygen exchange to occur and sufficient time for exhalation of CO_2.

Oxygen-Powered Breathing Devices

These manually triggered devices (e.g., demand valve) are not recommended for use in the pediatric patient because of the difficulty in regulating tidal volume and the amount of force used. Complications from these types of devices include gastric distention and trauma to the pulmonary and circulatory systems.

Endotracheal Intubation

When basic life-support methods of airway management have failed or the child needs complete immediate respiratory control, the method of choice is endotracheal intubation. Its advantages include the following:

- Complete and accurate airway control by visualizing the airway and placing the endotracheal tube directly into the lungs.
- Ability to suction the airway while protecting it from aspiration.
- A route for medications to be administered when IV access cannot be achieved.

The preferred method of intubation in the child is the endotracheal route. The nasotracheal route may cause massive hemorrhage or the tube may become obstructed by adenoid tissue. The blind nasotracheal method is not recommended, especially in children under 8 years of age, owing to the complexity of the anatomy in the child's nasal airway.

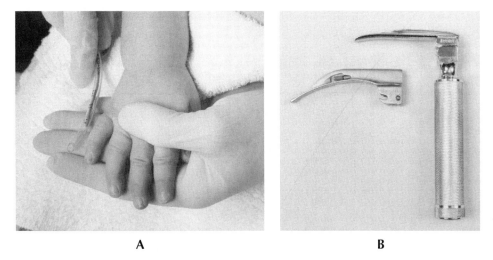

| A | B |

FIGURE 4.13   *(A) Selection of the correct-sized endotracheal tube. Note the vocal cord marking. Select a tube closest in size to the child's little finger. (B) Selection of a laryngoscope blade for intubation, either curved or straight and the appropriate size for the age of the child.*

Prior to the intubation attempt, select and prepare the equipment. Because of the child's small anatomy, some special considerations in equipment selection are important.

Children under 8 years of age should not be intubated with a cuffed tube. In infants and children, the cricoid ring is the site with the smallest diameter, not at the glottic area as in the adult. The cricoid ring will provide a natural and sufficient seal for the tube. The size of the tube used should be equal to the diameter of the little finger or external nares (Figure 4.13A). Have additional tubes one size smaller and one size larger available should they be needed.

The decision to use a curved or straight laryngoscope blade is one of preference and comfort. Use Table 4.1 as a guide for the size of the blade. After the blade has been selected, connect it to the laryngoscope handle and check the power and light source (Figure 4.13B).

Additional equipment to have available includes a bag-valve mask with reservoir and endotracheal tube, suction apparatus, and tape or one of the commercially available devices for securing the endotracheal tube.

The procedure for endotracheal intubation of infants and children is as follows:

- Preoxygenate the child with positive-pressure ventilation for 30 seconds prior to intubation.
- Place the child's head in a sniffing position, avoiding hyperextension of the neck because of the high, anterior position of the larynx. Place a folded towel under the child's shoulders to maintain neutral alignment of the airway and cervical spine. This padding is needed until about 8 years of age. Maintain in-line immobilization if cervical trauma is suspected (Figure 4.14).
- Time the length of the intubation effort. Each attempt should not exceed 30 seconds to prevent hypoxia and bradycardia. The child should be reoxygenated between attempts. Either hold your breath as you begin intubation or have someone keep time. When you need to take a breath, it is time to reoxygenate the patient.

TABLE 4.1 ■ *Guidelines for Appropriate Sizes of the Endotracheal Tube, Laryngoscope Blade, and Suction Catheter to Use in Infants and Children*

AGE	LARYNGOSCOPE BLADE	ENDOTRACHEAL TUBE	SUCTION CATHETER	DISTANCE (cm): MIDTRACHEA TO TEETH
Preterm	Miller 0	2.5 or 3.0	5 or 6 French	8
Newborn	Miller 0–1	3.0	6 French	10
6 Months	Miller 1	3.5	8 French	12
18 Months	Miller 1–2	4.0	8 French	13
3 Years	Miller 2	4.5	8 French	15
5 Years	Miller 2	5.0	10 French	16
6 Years	Miller 2	5.5	10 French	16
8 Years	Miller 2 Macintosh 2	6.0	10 French	18
12 Years	Macintosh 3	6.5	10 French	20
16 Years	Miller 3 Macintosh 3	7.0	12 French	22

Source: Adapted from "Pediatric Advanced Life Support," *JAMA,* 268(16): 2263, October 28, 1992, and Chameides, L. and Hazinski, M.F., eds. *Textbook of Pediatric Advanced Life Support,* 2nd ed. © American Heart Association, Dallas, TX, 1994. Used with permission.

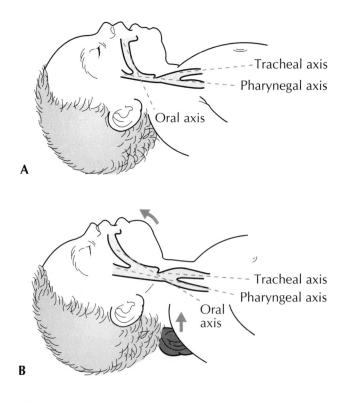

FIGURE 4.14 *Positioning the child before intubation. Note the relationships among the oral, tracheal, and pharyngeal axes (A) before and (B) after placing the child in neutral alignment, or sniffing position. Intubation is easier to accomplish when the axes are in close relationship with one another.*

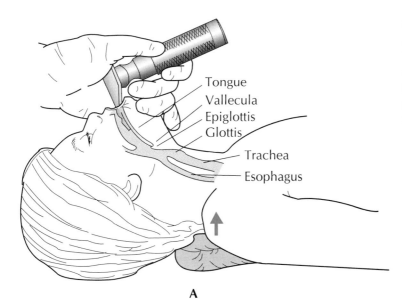

Tongue
Vallecula
Epiglottis
Glottis
Trachea
Esophagus

A

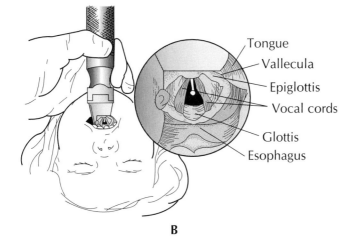

Tongue
Vallecula
Epiglottis
Vocal cords
Glottis
Esophagus

B

FIGURE 4.15 *Intubation of the child. Slowly insert the laryngoscope blade. To visualize the vocal cords, pull the handle upwards without touching the teeth. (A) Introduction of the laryngoscope. (B) Exposing the vocal cords and other internal anatomy.*

- Insert the laryngoscope blade to the right side of the mouth and sweep the tongue to the left side. Use a lifting motion to expose the vocal cords. The blade should not press on the teeth or gums of the maxilla (Figure 4.15A, B).
- Introduce the tube on the right side of the mouth. Pass the tube through the vocal cords to about 2–3 cm below the vocal cords. Confirm this by numbers on the tube or the double hatch marks on the distal end of the tube.
- Auscultate the chest to make sure the tube is in the trachea, not in the esophagus or in the right main stem bronchus. Listen at each lung apex and midaxillary area. Listen in the stomach area for gurgling associated with esophageal intubation. Signs of proper tube placement include:
  1. Augmented breath sounds on auscultation
  2. Condensation in the tube with exhalation
  3. Symmetrical bilateral chest wall movement with positive pressure ventilation
  4. Improved heart rate and color.

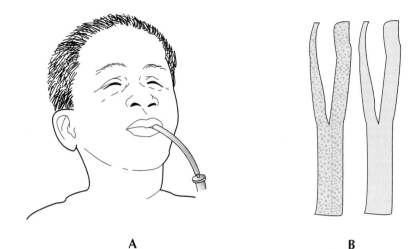

FIGURE 4.16 *(A) Once the endotracheal tube is in place, hold the tube to keep it from becoming dislodged. (B) Tear two strips of tape, each with a Y configuration. (C) Apply the tape across the maxillary area of the face, wrapping the lower half of the torn tape around the tube. (D) Repeat the taping with the second strip of tape, wrapping it around the tube in the opposite direction.*

- Tape the endotracheal tube securely to the child's face. Recheck the numbers on the tube at the mouth to make sure the position of the tube has not changed. Do not release the tube until the tape is securely attached (Figure 4.16A–D).
- Reconfirm the tube placement frequently, as the airway is short in infants, and minimal head movement may displace the tube. Consider maintaining neutral head position by placing towel rolls on each side of the child's head (Figure 4.17A–D).

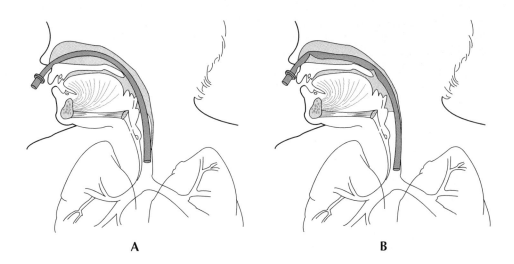

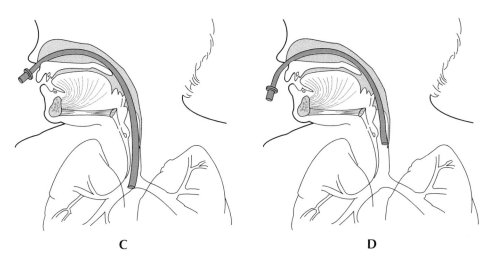

FIGURE 4.17 *Note possible endotracheal tube placements. (A) Ideal positioning in the trachea. (B) Kinked ET. (C) ET in right mainstem bronchus. (D) ET tube displaced against tracheal wall. Nasotracheal intubation was used in this case on a child over 8 years of age.*

Cricothyrotomy

Cricothyrotomy is a temporary life-saving procedure for an obstructed airway. It creates an opening through the cricothyroid membrane into the larynx. The procedure should only be used by trained personnel when all other procedures to open the airway fail. It is particularly difficult to perform in children, especially those under 3 years of age, because the airway is narrower, landmarks are less easily palpated, the infant's neck is short, the larynx is higher than an adult's, and the vocal cords are just above the cricothyroid membrane.

Indications for cricothyrotomy include the following:

- A child in respiratory or cardiac arrest with an obstructed airway
- Facial trauma with anatomic disruption that prevents other airway management
- All other methods of airway control have failed.

Cricothyrotomy should not be performed when there is an airway obstruction below the level of the cricoid cartilage; when there is a complete expiratory obstruction; when there is gross infection over puncture site; when there is a primary laryngeal injury; or when there is an inability to locate landmarks for puncture. Complications to the procedure include hypoxemia and CO_2 toxicity, esophageal perforation, subcutaneous emphysema, bleeding, infection, and damage to tracheal cartilage with possible vocal cord disruption.

The following equipment is needed to perform the cricothyrotomy: angiocath (14 or 16 gauge), a syringe filled with 1–2 cc of saline, an adapter to the infant endotracheal tube (size 3.0), oxygen, and a bag-valve mask with oxygen reservoir. Once the equipment is assembled, the following procedure may be used:

- Position child with slight neck extension, unless C-spine injury is suspected.
- Locate the cricothyroid and thyroid cartilages in the neck. The thyroid cartilage has a notch along the bottom edge, and the cricoid ring is the cartilage just beneath the thyroid cartilage (Figure 4.18).
- Once the thyroid notch is identified, move your fingers down to the cricothyroid membrane, between the two cartilages.
- Prepare the area with alcohol or other antiseptic solution.
- Insert the needle into the cricothyroid membrane at less than a 90° angle to the longitudinal axis of the neck. Maintain suction with the connected syringe until bubbles of air are noted in the saline. Then advance the catheter over the needle and reconfirm air flow with the syringe. Remove the needle.
- Attach the 3.0 endotracheal tube adapter to the hub of the catheter and begin ventilation with the bag mask.
- Secure the cannula with tape after confirming correct placement by auscultating for breath sounds over the lungs and stomach. Observe for kinking of the cannula.
- High-pressure oxygen should be provided (50 psi) for long-term ventilation because of the high resistance of the small tube.
- Bag-mask ventilation will give some time (about 40 minutes) until either intubation or a tracheostomy can be performed.
- If ventilation is inadequate, occlusion of the nose and mouth may decrease the upper airway leak.

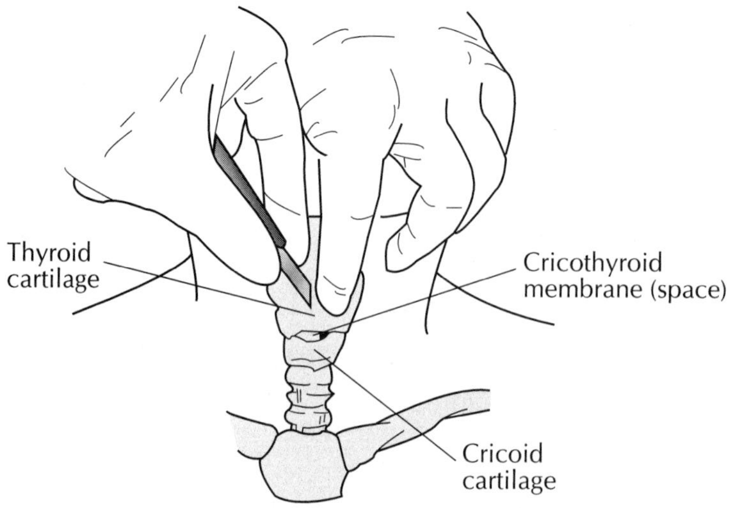

FIGURE 4.18 *Cricothyrotomy, location of the cricothyroid membrane for needle insertion.*

Thyroid cartilage

Cricothyroid membrane (space)

Cricoid cartilage

Chapter 4: Equipment and Procedures for Management of ABCs

Pleural Decompression

Tension pneumothorax develops following a chest injury that permits the progressive entry of air into the pleural space, elevating the pressure in the space above the atmospheric pressure level and causing the lung to collapse. The need for pleural (needle) decompression should be rapidly recognized and quickly performed by personnel experienced with this life-saving technique. See Chapters 9 and 11 for more details. Indications of the development of a tension pneumothorax and the need for pleural decompression include rapid deterioration in the child's heart rate, blood pressure, and perfusion (bradycardia, hypotension, delayed capillary refill, and decreased level of consciousness). Potential complications to this procedure include a collapsed lung if a pneumothorax is not present; trauma to the pulmonary artery or vena cava, resulting in hemothorax; and a lacerated lung.

The following equipment is needed for pleural decompression: An angiocath (14–18 gauge) and a flutter valve assembly. A McSwain dart or other special device may be used in older children, in place of an angiocath with flutter valves. The procedure for pleural decompression is as follows:

- Identify the side of the chest affected.
- Identify the landmarks for needle insertion. Use the 4th intercostal space at the level of the nipple line, along the anterior, midaxillary line for infants and young children. Use the 2nd intercostal space at the midclavicular line for older children (Figure 4.19).
- Prepare the skin with antiseptic.
- Advance the needle under the skin over the rib below the intercostal space selected and on into the intercostal space until air is expelled under pressure.
- Remove the needle and tape the catheter in place. The flutter valve should be attached, or connect the catheter to IV tubing and place it under water.
- Successful decompression is indicated by an immediate improvement in the child's heart rate, respiratory effort, blood pressure, and perfusion. If the child is being ventilated with a bag-valve mask, compliance will increase.

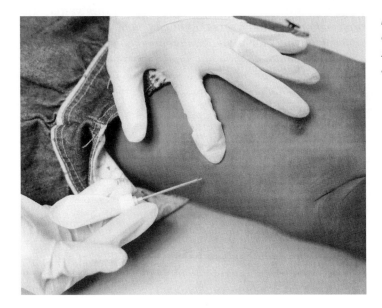

FIGURE 4.19 Location for needle thoracostomy is at the fourth or fifth intercostal space in the midaxillary line for infants and young children.

Establishing Intravenous Access

The decision to initiate intravenous (IV) therapy should be based on an assessment of the patient's immediate needs. This assessment should establish criteria that identify those patients that require immediate therapy, intermediate therapy, or no therapy. Below is a list of questions that should be considered before initiating therapy:

- What benefits will be gained from fluids or medications?
- How much time is involved in the procedure? Can it be safely performed en route?
- Is transport to the intended facility more appropriate?
- What is the rescuers' experience and skill level?
- How many resources will have to be committed to manage the patient? Will multiple personnel be required to restrain the child and initiate an IV?

While these criteria are not absolute, they are intended to be used as guidelines. When a decision has been made to establish IV therapy, it is essential for the rescuer to be familiar with the equipment and specific techniques to achieve IV access. Some tips for successful insertion include the following:

- Rubbing or patting the site may enhance local vein filling.
- Use warm packs to the area to enhance vein presentation.
- Elevate the lower extremities.
- Application of Pneumatic Anti-Shock Garment (PASG) and inflation of the leg compartments only may increase vein presentation in the upper extremities.

Sites

Select a site for intravenous access that will minimize the distance from the site to the central circulation. The larger and more central veins are choice sites. In the upper extremities consider using the cephalic, basilic, and median cubital veins of the forearm, as well as the median antecubital vein. In the lower extremities look for the great saphenous veins, the median marginal veins, and the veins of the dorsal arch. Avoid the fragile scalp veins that are inappropriate for resuscitation.

IV Equipment

Various types of equipment are used in establishing IV therapy. Thus, it is absolutely essential that the rescuer have a working knowledge of this equipment. In attempting to achieve IV placement in the pediatric patient, you will only make two attempts. Therefore, it is essential that you select the appropriate equipment for the job.

Types of Needless

The *butterfly* needle with attached catheter is supplied in sizes 25 to 16. It is used for establishing an IV line, using a scalp vein or for phlebotomy. The benefit of this device is its stability when it can be secured to the child's head. It is not recommended for peripheral lines, owing to infiltration from laceration of the vascular wall from extraneous movement of the rigid needle.

Over-the-needle catheters can be inserted in the back of the hands and feet, the antecubital fossa, and external jugular, saphenous, and femoral veins. These catheters range in size from 26 to 10. They are more difficult to insert but are much more likely to survive taping and patient movement.

The recommended IV solution for infants and children is Ringer's Lactate or Normal Saline for medical and trauma patients. These crystalloid solutions stay in the vascular space longer when compared to other solutions.

Antiseptic cleaner, saline, small syringe, small extension set, tape, and an arm board for immobilization are also required for IV therapy.

Establishing a Peripheral Line

The procedure for insertion of a peripheral line is as follows:

- Restrain the child, restricting as much movement of the IV site as possible.
- Place a rubber band tourniquet around the head for a scalp vein; a regular tourniquet for an extremity.
- Clean the skin with antiseptic and allow to dry.
- Check the patency of the catheter by injecting sterile saline through it with an attached 3-ml syringe and a small extension set.
- Stick the needle through the skin just below the vein and advance the needle toward the vein until flashback occurs. Try turning the bevel of the needle down in small children and infants. This approach prevents a puncture of the opposite vein wall before a flashback occurs. For angiocatheters, advance the catheter and pull out the needle.
- Remove the tourniquet and inject a small amount of saline into the vein to test for patency.
- Tape the needle in place and begin the infusion.

External Jugular Placement

Placement of an external jugular line in the pediatric patient should be used in cases where all other means of vascular access have failed and cervical spine injury is not suspected. There is the potential complication of puncture to the lung or great vessel because of the proximity of these structures to the neck. To insert a catheter into the external jugular vein, use the following technique:

- Place the child in a 20–30° Trendelenburg position with the head turned away from the side to be punctured. The right side is preferred.
- Restrain the child, restricting movement of the head and torso.
- Identify the external jugular vein and scrub the area with anticeptic.
- Insert an over-the-needle catheter into the vein for peripheral cannulation.
- When free blood flow is obtained, make sure that no air bubbles are in the tubing and attach the infusion set.

Umbilical Vein Cannulation

This method of establishing a lifeline should be used only in infants less than 5 days old. The procedure involves placing a catheter into the umbilical vein that leads directly into the liver. It should only be attempted by a rescuer who has been trained and is experienced in the procedure. The following equipment is required for this procedure: a scalpel blade; a 5.0 French umbilical catheter; feeding tube, or a 14–20-gauge angiocath; and a 3-way stopcock and sterile saline-filled syringe.

The procedure for umbilical vein cannulation includes the following:

- Trim the cord to 1–2 cm above the skin attachment and hold it firmly to prevent bleeding. A piece of umbilical tape can be tied around the umbilical stump to control bleeding.
- The umbilical vein is identified as the single thin-wall vessel. The arteries are paired, thick-wall vessels.

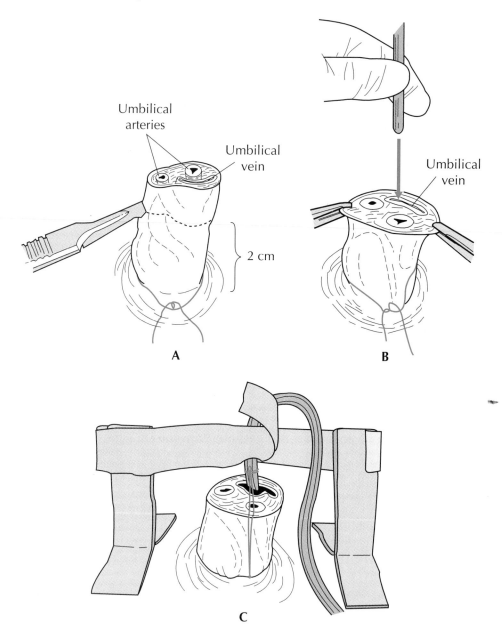

FIGURE 4.20   Umbilical vein cannulation procedure. (A) Identify the umbilical vein after trimming the cord. (B) Insert an umbilical catheter or angiocath into the vein, advancing the tip just until blood return is apparent. (C) Place a tie around the base of the cord to hold the catheter in place. Stabilize the catheter with tape as illustrated and begin IV infusion.

- Attach the umbilical catheter or angiocatheter filled with saline to a stopcock. Advance the catheter so the tip is just below the surface of the skin, just until blood return is apparent. Insert the catheter no further so as to avoid infusion directly into the liver.
- If there is no free blood flow, then the catheter is most likely wedged against the liver and should be pulled back some until free flow occurs.
- Place a tie around the umbilical stump to hold the catheter in place and prevent bleeding. Attach the IV and begin infusion. Tape the catheter and tubing to the child's stomach (Figure 4.20A–C).

Intraosseous Infusion

The technique of intraosseous infusion was first described 70 years ago. It was used extensively in the 1930s and 1940s for administration of fluids and blood. It has gained renewed widespread use in emergency resuscitation over the past 14 years. The major advantage of the intraosseous (IO) infusion is that the bone shaft acts as a noncollapsible vein through which medication and fluids can be administered. While the IO technique is a proven means of establishing a lifeline, it should not be the first choice.

Indications for IO insertion include the following:

- Attempts at establishing a peripheral line have failed. As a rule the rescuers are allowed 3 attempts or 90 seconds.
- Drugs and fluids need to be given to a child with unstable vital signs who is unconscious or unresponsive.
- The child is under 6 years of age, although IO infusion is now performed on older children.

Equipment to have available for IO infusion includes Betadine, disposable gloves, adhesive tape, gauze 4 × 4s, a 10-cc syringe, a 15–19-gauge bone marrow needle or 18–20 gauge short spinal needle with a stylet. The procedure for establishing an intraosseous line is as follows:

- Place the infant or child in a supine position.
- Identify and locate the bony landmarks. The preferred site is the proximal tibia, 1 to 2 finger breadths below the tibial tuberosity on the anteromedial surface (Figure 4.21A). An alternate site is 1–2 cm proximal to the medial malleolus on the anteromedial surface of the distal tibia.
- Prep the site with Betadine.
- Direct and insert the needle, with the stylet in place, perpendicular to the bone or angled away from the joint, avoiding the epiphyseal plate. Insert with pressure and in a boring motion until penetration into the bone marrow, which is marked by a sudden lack of resistance.
- Remove the stylet and attach the syringe with stopcock. If the needle is properly placed in the bone marrow, aspiration of blood with marrow may be possible, but does not always occur. Another sign of proper placement is lack of resistance to infusion and no sign of infiltration. The needle stands without support (Figure 4.21B).
- Attach the IV tubing. A pressure bag or 60-ml syringe with a stopcock setup is needed to infuse fluids.
- Stabilize the needle on both sides with sterile gauze and secure with tape (Figure 4.21C).

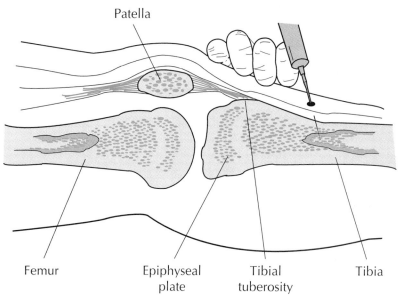

Patella

Femur   Epiphyseal   Tibial   Tibia
         plate   tuberosity

A

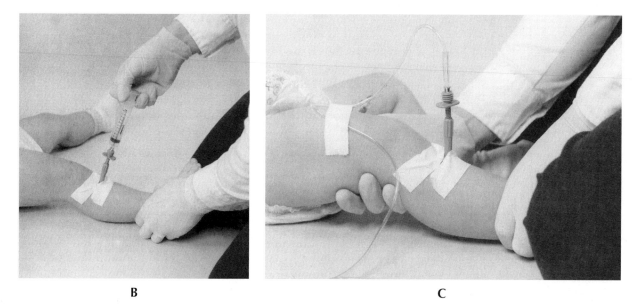

B   **C**

FIGURE 4.21   Intraosseous infusion technique. (A) Locate the site for intraosseous needle insertion, two fin-ger breadths below the tibial tuberosity on the anteromedial surface of the tibia. Insert the needle at an angle toward the foot. (B) After needle insertion, attach a syringe with saline to the needle. Try to aspirate blood from the marrow or infuse a small amount of saline through to the needle. No resistance to infusion should be noted. (C) Tape the needle and IV catheter for stabilization during transport.

Pneumatic Anti-Shock Garment

The use of the Pneumatic Anti-Shock Garment (PASG) has engendered much controversy in the field of emergency medicine. Although many studies have assessed the effectiveness of this piece of equipment, the question still remains as to its benefit and where, if at all, it should be used in augmenting circulation in children. The 1994 National Standard Curriculum for EMT-Bs does not recommend the use of PASG in children.

Local medical direction must provide guidance in this therapy. The advantages that have been demonstrated by the use of PASG in adults are:

- Increased peripheral vascular resistance.
- Improvement of blood flow to the heart, lungs, and brain.
- Tamponading effect to areas underneath the garment.

The PASG cannot and should not be used as a long-term support device; its use constitutes a life-saving, hemorrhage controlling, short-term technique. Use of the PASG in pediatric patients should be initiated only when local medical direction recommends it.

Application Criteria

The systolic blood pressure reading is the criteria used for application and inflation of the PASG. Place the garment on the child when the systolic blood pressure is less than 80 mm Hg and when signs of shock are present (tachycardia, pallor, diaphoresis, delayed capillary refill time). Do NOT inflate it until consultation with medical direction or the patient's systolic blood pressure drops to under 60 mm Hg.

Inflate the leg compartments only (Figure 4.22). The abdominal compartment is only inflated in the presence of a pelvic fracture and hemorrhage. The pressure placed against the abdomen may cause the diaphragm to stop functioning, resulting in ventilatory compromise and respiratory arrest. The trousers are inflated adequately when the Velcro attachments begin to separate. Monitor the patient's vital signs. Application of the PASG in children is no different from the procedure used for adults.

Defibrillation and Synchronized Cardioversion

Defibrillation is the untimed depolarization of cardiac cells that allows a spontaneous organized heart beat to return. The same principle is used in cardioversion, but in that case the charge delivered is timed.

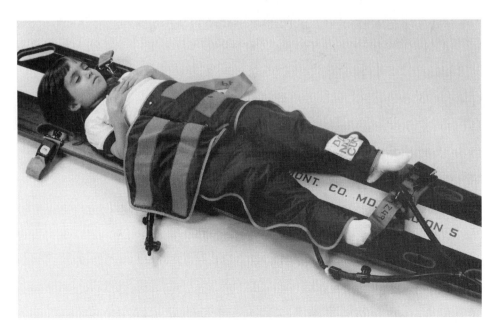

FIGURE 4.22 Application of Pneumatic Anti-Shock Garment (PASG).

The exact paddle size needed for children or different body size is not currently known. As a rule, the electrode or paddle that covers the largest area of the chest is the correct size. The paddles or electrodes should have a space between them to allow for conduction. The position of the paddles should be below the right clavicle and just below the left nipple, more lateral than medial. In small children, the one paddle may be placed on the anterior chest and the other on the posterior chest with the heart between them (Figure 4.23).

Defibrillation

The sequence for defibrillation should be as follows:

- Continue CPR with as little interruption as possible.
- Apply conductive gel to the appropriately sized paddles or place pediatric defibrillation pads on the chest.
- Turn the defibrillator on and check to see that it is not in the synchronous mode.
- Select the energy dose and charge the capacitor (2 J/kg).
- Stop chest compressions and place the paddles in the proper position.
- Recheck the rhythm.
- Clear the area to ensure that no personnel are in direct contact with the patient.
- Apply firm pressure to the paddles while depressing both discharge buttons simultaneously.
- Reassess the rhythm and pulse. If ventricular fibrillation (VF) persists, repeat countershock at twice the initial dose (4 J/kg). If an organized rhythm has been established, check the pulses and continue CPR as needed. If VF recurs, immediately repeat the countershock, using the same dose.

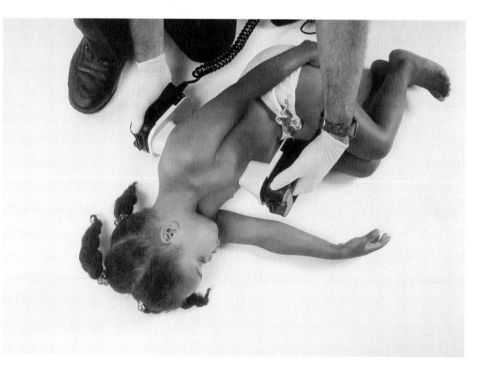

FIGURE 4.23 *Anterior-posterior placement of defibrillator paddles.*

This procedure is the same as that outlined for defibrillation except as follows:

- If the paddles are the monitor type, the ECG must be connected to a defibrillator.
- The synchronizer circuit must be activated.
- The discharge buttons must be held until the countershock is delivered.
- Initial dose of energy is 0.5 J/kg.
- Reassess the ECG and pulse.
- If a second shock is required, double the dose.

Spinal Immobilization

The objective of spinal immobilization is to protect the injured spinal column from further injury. This can be achieved in a variety of ways and with a wide array of equipment. Because every situation is unique, it is not the intent to address every conceivable possibility. Therefore, general guidelines will be presented.

- Select the appropriate equipment for the situation. This includes cervical collars, immobilization devices, and all other equipment designed or routinely used on children.
- Assess the scene for safety of the rescuer and the child.
- Assess the ABCs and treat accordingly.
- Apply manual stabilization.
- Measure and apply the appropriate-sized cervical collar. The correct-sized collar should limit the amount of cervical movement. Most commercial cervical collars are not sized for children under 24 months of age.
- Select the appropriate immobilization device, a pediatric immobilizer, long board, Kendricks Extrication Device (KED), etc. This device should limit the majority of body movement. This is not easily achieved unless matched with an equally limiting strapping device or system. Papoose-type boards are not appropriate for immobilization (Figure 4.24A–D).
- When immobilizing children, they will not sit still to allow you to place a device on them. Skill, patience, and practice are all necessary to achieve success.

References for Management of ABCs

Brownstein, D., et al., "Prehospital endotracheal intubation of children by paramedics," *Annals of Emergency Medicine,* 28, no. 1 (July 1996), pp. 34–39.

Chameides, L., and Hazinski, M.F., ed., *Textbook of Pediatric Advanced Life Support,* 2nd ed. Dallas: American Heart Association, 1994.

Eichelberger, M., Stossel-Pratsch, G., eds., *Pediatric Emergencies Manual.* Rockville, MD: Aspen Publishing Co., 1984, pp. 13–31.

Luten, R.C., Wears, R.L., Broselow, J., et. al., "Length based endotracheal tube and emergency equipment in pediatrics," *Annals of Emergency Medicine,* 21 (August 8, 1992), pp. 900–904.

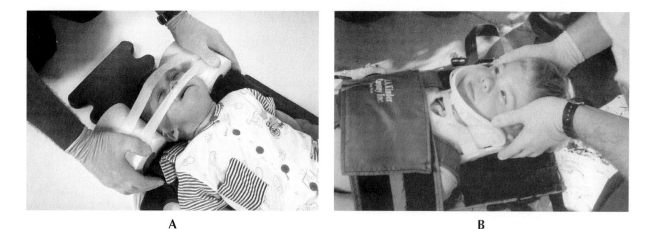

A   B

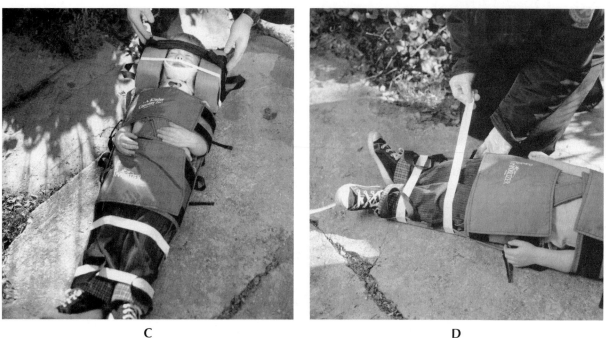

C   D

FIGURE 4.24   *Spinal immobilization techniques. (A) Immobilize the infant's head with a towel roll and tape across the forehead and maxilla. (B) Cervical collars can be used in older children. (C) Immobilization of a child on a pediatric immobilizer. (D) Restraint of the legs: Use tape across the knees and lower legs.*

Moront, M., Williams, J., Eichelberger, M.R., et. al., "The injured child, an approach to care," *Pediatric Clinics of North America,* 41, no. 6, (December 1994), pp. 1201–1224.

Reynolds, T., and Jones, T.R., "Pediatric airway," *Emergency,* 28, no. 4 (April 1996), pp. 42–47.

Rusconi, F., Castagneto, M., Gagliard, L., et. al., "Reference values for respiratory rates in the first 3 years of life," *Pediatrics,* 94, no. 3 (September 1994), pp. 350–354.

Pediatric Cardiopulmonary Resuscitation

OBJECTIVES

When you have completed this chapter you should be able to

▶ Identify the most frequent causes of cardiac arrest in the newborn, infant, and child.
▶ Describe the technique for ventilations and compressions in CPR for the following age groups:
  • newborns
  • infants
  • children
▶ Describe signs that indicate CPR is effective in the pediatric patient.
▶ List the steps in the procedure to relieve airway obstruction for infants and children.
▶ Describe appropriate management of specific conditions leading to cardiac arrest in children with foreign body airway obstruction.

Overview of Respiratory and Cardiac Arrest in Children

The child's heart is generally healthy and strong, undamaged by smoking and dietary abuse. Cardiac arrest in children is usually the result of progressive deterioration in respiratory and cardiac status, rather than a sudden event. The usual sequence is a long period of hypoxia, resulting in respiratory arrest. Without intervention, full cardiopulmonary arrest occurs.

Because there is a long period of hypoxia, and accompanying metabolic acidosis and tissue damage, the resuscitation of children who have progressed to cardiac arrest is frequently unsuccessful by both prehospital or hospital providers. Thus, it is important to identify infants and children with respiratory compromise and intervene early. Provision of adequate support for respiratory failure will often prevent respiratory arrest.

In children common causes of hypoxia that result in cardiac arrest include the following:

- Airway obstruction from a foreign body, infection, or congenital defect
- Trauma
- Asphyxia from suffocation, drowning, or smoke inhalation
- Sudden infant death syndrome

Other causes of cardiopulmonary arrest in children include:

- Untreated or undertreated hypoperfusion (shock) that results in hypoxia and tissue damage; shock may occur with burns, severe dehydration, blood loss, sepsis, and anaphylaxis;
- Metabolic disorders involving an electrolyte imbalance such as that associated with dehydration from vomiting and diarrhea;
- Poisoning by a central nervous system depressant, which decreases the respiratory rate to the point of hypoxia and apnea;
- Congenital heart defects or acquired heart disease.

Respiratory Failure and Ventilatory Failure

Respiratory distress, preceding respiratory failure, occurs when the child attempts to compensate for hypoxia by increasing the work of breathing. Signs include tachypnea, retractions, nasal flaring, and tachycardia. If

FIGURE 5.1   *Progression of Ventilatory Failure to Cardiac Arrest*

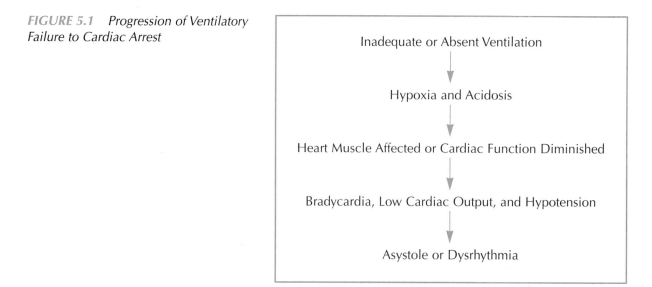

Inadequate or Absent Ventilation

↓

Hypoxia and Acidosis

↓

Heart Muscle Affected or Cardiac Function Diminished

↓

Bradycardia, Low Cardiac Output, and Hypotension

↓

Asystole or Dysrhythmia

Chapter 5: Pediatric Cardiopulmonary Resuscitation

hypoxia is not managed (e.g., by supplemental oxygen), the carbon dioxide tension in the blood increases, leading to metabolic acidosis and respiratory failure.

Respiratory failure results from prolonged impairment of pulmonary gas exchange in which there is inadequate oxygenation of the blood and inadequate elimination of carbon dioxide, such as due to poor gas exchange.

Ventilatory failure results when an infant or a child tires from the increased work of breathing. The child does not have the ability to sustain a rapid respiratory rate for lengthy periods and will begin breathing ineffectively at a lower rate that eventually leads to respiratory arrest and bradycardia. Cardiac arrest will result if intervention does not occur rapidly. Other causes of a slow respiratory rate include hypothermia and poisoning by a central nervous system depressant (Figure 5.1).

History

Important information to obtain during the history includes the following:

S How long has the child been experiencing breathing difficulties? Has the child been coughing or have any cold symptoms? Have the symptoms been getting better or worse?

A Does the child have any allergies?

M Does the child take any medications? Has the child taken any medications for this condition?

P Has the child ever had an asthma attack? Has the child recently had a respiratory infection (cold, croup, pneumonia) or any other lung condition? Has the child ever been treated by a doctor for a similar breathing difficulty?

L When did the child last eat or drink? What did the child have to eat (peanuts, raisins, grapes, hard candy, hot dogs)?

E Could the child have possibly choked on something (like a small toy, object, or food item)? Has the child sustained any recent injuries (head injury, chest injury, or hypoperfusion)? How long ago did it happen?

Assessment

You should recognize the potential for respiratory failure in the child with diminishing level of responsiveness, respiratory rate over 60 per minute, mottled or cyanotic color, and poor muscle tone. This is a child in need of rapid intervention to prevent further deterioration to ventilatory failure and respiratory arrest. A decreasing respiratory rate of less than 20 per minute may be an indicator of ventilatory failure, especially when no intervention has been provided for respiratory distress (Table 5.1).

Management

Basic life support (BLS) management for respiratory and ventilatory failure includes the following steps:

- Monitor the airway, ventilations, the circulatory status, and mental status, including vital signs and body temperature.
- Maintain the child with respiratory distress in a position of comfort. The child will generally find the best position to maintain the airway.
- Administer high-flow, high-concentration oxygen by face mask.
- Do not create any additional anxiety in the child with invasive procedures. Do not inspect the mouth or tongue with a tongue blade.
- Transport rapidly.

TABLE 5.1 ■ *Signs of Respiratory and Ventilatory Failure*

RESPIRATORY FAILURE	VENTILATORY FAILURE
Altered mental status	Altered mental status to unresponsive
Tachycardia	Tachycardia to bradycardia
Tachypnea, greater than 60 per minute	Respiratory rate below lowest normal rate for age
Weak, limp	Weak, limp
Retractions	Retractions
Mottled or cyanotic color	Mottled or cyanotic color
Head bobbing with each breath	
Diminished breath sounds	Diminished breath sounds
Weak central pulses	Weak central pulses
Absent peripheral pulses	Absent peripheral pulses

CAUTION!

> If the child's respiratory rate is greater than 60/min, and oxygen alone does not result in a lower respiratory rate, it may be necessary to assist ventilation with a bag-valve mask, using high-flow, high-concentration oxygen at a rate slightly higher than the child is breathing. Once you have control of the child's ventilations with the bag-valve mask, begin slowing the manual ventilation rate to less than 60/min. Then maintain the ventilation rate at 40–45/min.
>
> If the respiratory rate begins decreasing, and the child's mental status deteriorates, assist ventilations (by bag mask with high-concentration oxygen). Maintain ventilations at 35–40/min and monitor the patient's vital signs.

Advanced life support (ALS) treatment additionally will include:

- Endotracheal intubation,
- Establishing a peripheral IV line with Ringer's Lactate or Normal Saline at a keep-open rate. Transport should not be unnecessarily delayed to accomplish this, and
- Administering medications according to local protocols.

Rescue Breathing

If the child is found to be unresponsive, shake patient gently to determine the level of response. Protect the cervical spine if trauma is suspected. Call for additional help if the child is not breathing. Position the child with the head in neutral alignment, or sniffing position prior to opening the airway. Make sure you do not hyperextend the neck. (Refer to Figure 4.1, page 49).

The muscles in the mouth and throat will relax when the child is unresponsive, allowing the tongue to fall back into the throat and to occlude the airway. Manually open the airway with either the chin-lift or jaw-thrust maneuver. The tongue will follow the mandible forward to open the airway. The modified jaw-thrust maneuver should be used with both hands, keeping the neck stabilized whenever a cervical spine injury is suspected. When the airway cannot be maintained or a good seal is not achieved with one-rescuer ventilation, have one rescuer secure the airway while the other rescuer ventilates.

Once the airway is opened, check again for breathing. Place your ear close to the child's nose and mouth, listening and feeling for exhaled air flow (Figure 5.2). Look at the chest and abdomen for movement. If there is no obvious spontaneous breathing, begin rescue breathing or manual ventilation.

Use mouth-to-mask breathing (mouth-to-mouth if no mask is available to fit the child) for children. If mouth-to-mouth ventilation is performed, pinch the patient's nose tightly. For infants, use the mouth-to-mouth and nose technique (Figure 5.3). Give two *slow* breaths (1 to 1.5 seconds/breath) to keep the pressure low and avoid gastric distention. Use enough pressure and volume to make the chest rise. The rate of rescue breathing, when chest compressions are not performed, should closely approximate the normal respiratory rate of the child. Rates are shown below:

- Newborns—40–60/min, every 1 to $1^{1}/_{2}$ seconds
- Infants—20/min, every 3 seconds
- Children—20/min, every 3 seconds

When performing rescue breathing or assisted ventilation, the inspiratory and expiratory phases should be equal in length, a 1:1 ratio. One technique to use to obtain the correct rhythm is the "Waltz Method." The first count is for inspiration and the second and third counts are for expiration. To get the correct rhythm, say Breathe - 2 - 3, Breathe - 2 - 3,…. The time it takes to say "Breathe" should equal the time it takes to say 2, 3. Then get the correct rate for the ventilation.

The rescuer can increase the oxygen concentration delivered during rescue breathing from 16% to 28% by wearing nasal prongs with oxygen flowing at 10 l/min. As soon as possible, switch to a bag-valve mask with an oxygen reservoir to continue manual ventilation of the child. The size

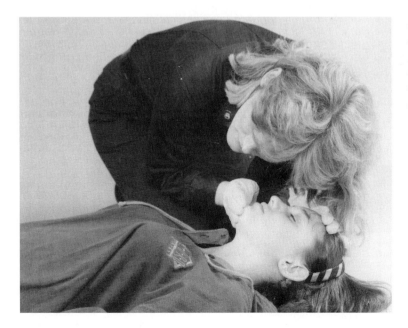

FIGURE 5.2 *Assess for breathing after opening the airway by placing your ear close to the child's nose and mouth. While you listen and feel for exhaled air, look at the patient's chest and abdomen for movement.*

FIGURE 5.3 *Use the mouth-to-mouth and nose technique of rescue breathing for infants. Use nasal cannula to increase oxygen delivery to the infant.*

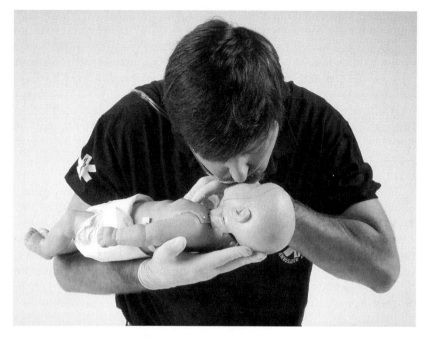

and seal of the mask are crucial. The ALS provider will want to consider intubation if spontaneous breathing does not resume quickly.

If there is a high resistance to airflow and the chest does not rise, assume there is an airway obstruction. Reposition the child's head with the chin-lift or jaw-thrust maneuver. If there is still an obstruction, suspect an occlusion by a foreign body and reattempt ventilation. See guidelines for airway obstruction management (pp. 83–86). Once the first two breaths have been successfully given, check for the presence of a pulse. The brachial pulse is recommended for infants because their neck is short, making the carotid pulse difficult to palpate. Children over 1 year of age can have their carotid or brachial pulse palpated (Figure 5.4). If the pulse is absent, initiate chest compressions. If a pulse is present, continue rescue breathing, checking for the presence of a pulse periodically.

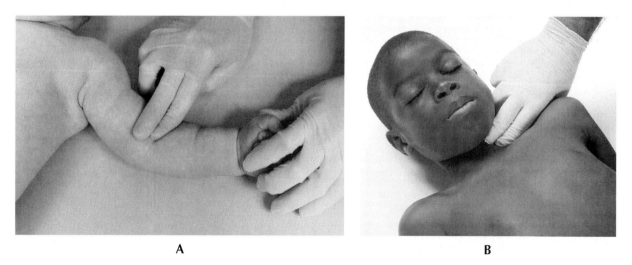

A   **B**

FIGURE 5.4   Palpate the pulse after breathing for the child. (A) Assess the brachial pulse in infants and young children. (B) Assess the carotid pulse in children over 1 year of age.

Chest Compressions

Chest compressions are indicated when there is no central pulse palpated or there is a pulse rate less than 60 beats/min or between 60 and 80 beats/min that is not increasing rapidly after adequate airway measures in newborns; less than 80 beats/min in infants; or less than 60 beats/min in children (bradycardia) unresponsive to ventilation and oxygenation (Table 5.2).

When initiating CPR, make sure the child is supine on a hard surface. Hand position for performing compressions varies with the age of the child (Figure 5.5).

- *Newborns.* Place both thumbs on the sternum just below the imaginary line across the nipples, with the fingers around the torso, supporting the back. This hand position requires an additional rescuer to provide ventilation. When an extra rescuer in unavailable, the hand position used for the infant is also effective.
- *Infants.* Position the hand by placing the index finger of the hand farthest from the infant's head just below the nipple line on the sternum. The area of compression is 1 finger breadth below this imaginary line, at the location of the middle and ring fingers. Make sure the fingers are not on the xiphoid.
- *Children over 1 year of age.* Position the hand by following with your index and middle finger the rib cage margin to the notch where the ribs and sternum meet. Place the middle finger in this notch with the index finger next to it. Visually identify the position of the index finger and place the heel of the same hand next to it, with the long axis of the heel parallel to that of the sternum.
- *Children over 8 years of age.* Position the hands as you do for children over 1 year of age. Use both hands interlocked for compressions.

Chest compressions should be smooth rather than jerky. Allow the chest to resume normal position without removing the fingers or hand from the sternum. Develop a compression-relaxation rhythm with equal time for each. Both the rate and the depth of compressions vary with the age of the child.

Compressions must be coordinated with rescue breathing. A 3:1 compression to ventilation ratio should be used for newborns. At the end of every fifth compression, a pause (of no more than 1 second) should be allowed for ventilation. A 5:1 compression-to-ventilation ratio should be maintained for both infants and children: 20 breaths/min for infants and children. Reassess the child after 20 full cycles (approximately 1 minute) and every few minutes after that. Controversy continues regarding the adequacy of this rate of ventilation, especially with infants and small children who are already hypoxic. However, achieving the optimal number of chest compressions and allowing 1 second for each ventilation is not an easily accomplished task.

TABLE 5.2 ■ *Rate and Depth of Chest Compressions for Children of Different Ages*

Age	Rate	Depth*
Newborns	120/min	0.5–0.75 inch
Infants	at least 100/min	0.5–1.0 inch ($^1/_3$ to $^1/_2$ depth of chest)
Children (1–8 years)	100/min	1.0–1.5 inches (1 to $1^1/_2$ depth of chest)
Children (over 8)	100/min	1.5–2.0 inches

*Make sure femoral or brachial pulses are periodically checked to assure adequate chest compressions.

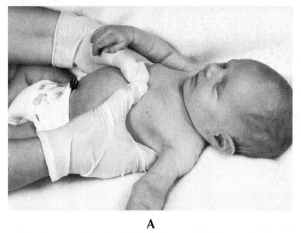

A
Newborns: Use both thumbs and light pressure.

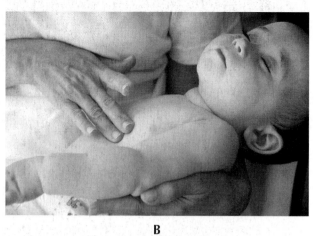

B
Infants: Use tips of fingures and light pressure.

FIGURE 5.5   Positioning the hands for chest compressions differs according to the age and size of the child. (A) Newborn, (B) Infant, (C) Children between 1 and 8 years of age. (Parts B and C reproduced with permission from Grant et al. Emergency Care, Fifth Ed., © 1990 Prentice Hall.)

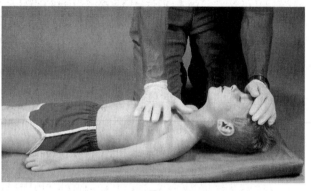

C
Children: Use heel of one hand only.

When there is only one rescuer, even more compromises are necessary to coordinate compressions and ventilation. If the rescuer hopes to provide the optimal number of compressions and ventilations each minute, time is inadequate either to move the hand from the chest for the chin-lift or to physically identify the landmarks for compression after each ventilation.

■ In infants, a head-tilt should be used *without the chin-lift* to maintain airway patency after the initial two ventilations. The rescuer should observe the patient's chest to make sure it rises with each breath, repositioning the patient's head if chest rise is not apparent.
■ In children the chin-lift and head-tilt are both needed to maintain an open airway for ventilations. The hand performing the compressions must be used for the chin-lift, and then be returned to the chest position for compressions using only visual recall of position.

Signs of effective CPR include the following:

■ Brachial or femoral pulses are felt during compressions.
■ The heart resumes beating, and there is a palpable spontaneous pulse.
■ There is improved color as the child pinks up.
■ There is spontaneous movement of the arms and legs.
■ There are spontaneous respiratory efforts, such as gasping with chest rise.
■ The pupils constrict to light.

Management of Parents

When a child needs CPR, the parent is in crisis. It is important to be gentle, but firm, with the parent so you can proceed with resuscitation. Parents will be most reassured if you demonstrate how you are helping the child and convey control of the situation. When available, another pre-hospital provider, police, family member, or bystander should be employed to support the parent. If no one is available, it may be helpful to enlist the parent's support in caring for the child. Direct the parent to perform simple tasks (get the child's favorite toy or the parent's own wallet or purse in preparation for the trip to the hospital). Remember, any instructions you give should be clear and brief. *Parents will tend to hear the instructions but not listen to them.* Anxiety also produces a short-term memory loss, so instructions will usually need repeating.

Airway Obstruction

Aspiration of a foreign body is a common problem in children under 3 years of age. In 1992 it was the third leading cause of unintentional injury deaths in infants between 1 month and 1 year of age (12.6% of this age group) and the fourth leading cause of unintentional injury deaths in children 1 to 4 years of age (3.9% in this age group). However, many more such events occurred that did not result in death.

Infants and young children explore the environment by putting objects such as pins, coins, and parts of toys in their mouth. They also have few or no teeth and have yet to develop full control of swallowing. For this reason, foods are often aspirated as well. Commonly aspirated foods include hot dogs, peanuts, grapes, and candy. Their size, shape, and consistency contribute to greater severity of symptoms. If the object is large enough, complete occlusion of the airway can occur.

History

Important information to obtain upon arrival:

S   Did the child have a sudden episode of coughing, choking, wheezing, and cyanosis that was observed by a care provider? Is the child still coughing or choking? Is there any physical evidence present? Was this sudden onset of respiratory distress associated with an illness?

A   Does the child have any known allergies?

M   Does the child take any medications? If yes, for what health problem?

P   Does the child have any known respiratory condition? Does the child have any problems with swallowing?

L   When did the child eat? What foods were eaten (any foods like grapes, hot dogs, peanuts, hard candy)?

E   Was this episode associated with eating any particular food or did it occur with play activities?

Assessment

The child who has aspirated a foreign object may be in any stage of respiratory distress. During the initial assessment (primary survey), note the ability of the child to talk, cry, cough, or wheeze. In this case the child has a partial obstruction. The child may also be unresponsive with no spontaneous breathing, in which case there may be total occlusion of the airway. Infections, such as croup and epiglottitis, also cause airway obstruction, but the onset is longer, over hours or days. Management of airway obstruction for these infections is outlined in Chapter 6.

Management

BLS management for an *incomplete* airway obstruction is the same as that for a child with respiratory failure.

■ Permit the child to find the best position to keep the airway open, and maintain the child in that position.
■ Encourage the child to cough.
■ Administer high-flow, high-concentration oxygen by nonrebreather face mask if the child will tolerate it.
■ Do not create any additional anxiety in the child by performing invasive procedures.
■ Transport immediately and rapidly.
■ Attempt to open the child's airway if the child's coughing becomes ineffective or if there is increased respiratory difficulty accompanied by stridor.

Attempts to clear the occluded airway should be made when the aspiration of a foreign body was witnessed or strongly suspected in the following cases:

■ There is a responsive child who cannot talk or cry.
■ There is a nonresponsive, nonbreathing child after usual attempts to open the airway are unsuccessful.

BLS management for the **infant** with an *obstructed airway* includes the following steps (Figure 5.6):

■ Perform a series of 5 back blows and 5 chest thrusts. (The Heimlich maneuver is not recommended because of the potential for intra-abdominal injury.)

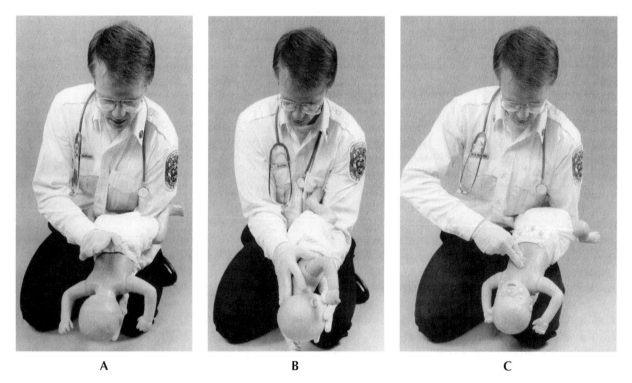

| A | B | C |

FIGURE 5.6 *Management of an obstructed airway in infant. (A) Perform 5 back blows with the infant face down, head lower than the body. (B) Turn the infant face upward, sandwiched between both of your arms. (C) Perform 5 chest thrusts.*

1. Position the infant face down, with the head lower than the body, on one arm.
2. Use one hand to deliver 5 forceful blows between the shoulder blades of the back.
3. Sandwich the infant between both arms and turn the patient's face upwards. Support the infant on your thigh with the head lower than the body.
4. Deliver 5 chest thrusts in the same location where chest compressions are performed.

■ Open the airway with the tongue-jaw lift and look for the foreign body. Remove any foreign material observed. Make *NO* blind finger sweeps in the mouth; this could cause the foreign body to be pushed back even farther into the airway.
■ If no spontaneous breathing is observed, perform rescue breathing. If the airway is still obstructed, repeat the sequence of back blows, chest thrusts, inspection of the mouth, and rescue breathing until the airway obstruction is removed.
■ Transport patient rapidly to the nearest hospital.

BLS management for the **child** with an *obstructed airway* includes the following steps (Figure 5.7):

■ Use subdiaphragmatic abdominal thrusts (the Heimlich maneuver).
■ When the child is conscious, perform this maneuver standing behind the child who is sitting or standing:
1. Make a fist with one hand, placing the thumb side against the middle of the child's abdomen, slightly above the navel.
2. Grasp the fist with the other hand and press into the child's abdomen with a quick upward thrust. Take care not to press on the xiphoid or the rib cage.

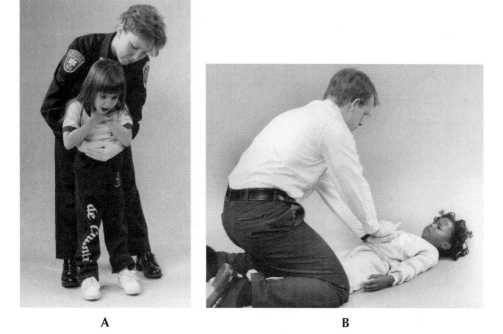

A   B

FIGURE 5.7   Management of an obstructed airway in the child. (A) Perform subdiaphragmatic abdominal thrusts when the child is conscious and sitting or standing. (B) Straddle the unconscious child and perform abdominal thrusts.

- When the child is unconscious and lying on the floor:
  1. Position yourself at the child's feet or straddle the child.
  2. Place the heel of one hand in the middle of the child's abdomen above the navel. Place the other hand on top of the first and press the abdomen in the midline with quick upward thrusts.
- Individual thrusts should continue until the foreign body is expelled or 5 abdominal thrusts have been delivered.
- Check for the foreign body in the mouth and remove it if seen. *Caution:* NO BLIND FINGER SWEEPS.
- Check for spontaneous breathing and if not present, attempt to perform rescue breathing. If no ventilation is possible, repeat the sequence until the airway is open or the child loses consciousness.
- Transport patient rapidly to the nearest hospital.

Common Pediatric Dysrhythmias

Bradycardia

This is the most common dysrhythmia in children. It usually develops as a result of hypoxia, hypotension, and acidosis. Bradycardia also develops with vagal stimulation, caused by suctioning or intubation that is too aggressive without adequate reoxygenation. The newborn will become apneic and then hypoxic if cold oxygen is directed to the infant's face in the distribution of the trigeminal nerve (mammalian diving reflex).

Assessment

The child will have signs of hypoxia and a slower heart rate than expected for his or her age (less than 60/min in infants and children under 8 years of age). Poor systemic perfusion may be present. The rhythm strip will show a slow rate; the P wave may or may not be present; the QRS duration may be normal or prolonged; and the P and QRS waves are often unrelated (Figure 5.8).

Management

BLS management for bradycardia includes the following:

- Control the airway.
- Give high-flow, high-concentration oxygen and ventilatory support to prevent progression to asystole.
- Assist ventilations prior to respiratory arrest with a bag-valve mask and high-concentration, high-flow oxygen; hyperventilate. Make inspiratory and expiratory phases of each breath equal in length.
- Initiate CPR if the child is unresponsive and the heart rate is less than 80/min in infants or 60/min in young children when there is no response to ventilation with high-concentration oxygen.
- Keep the patient warm.
- Provide immediate and rapid transport to the hospital.

The ALS provider should additionally initiate the following care:

- Attach a cardiac monitor and record a rhythm strip.
- Begin endotracheal intubation.
- Establish an IV or intraosseous line. Do not delay transport to establish the line.

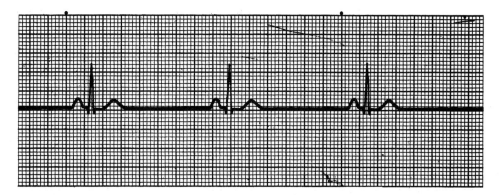

FIGURE 5.8   Rhythm strip indicating bradycardia in the child with a rate of 40 per minute.

- Epinephrine and atropine administered by endotracheal tube or IV may be ordered by medical direction or protocols, when oxygen and ventilation do not restore the heart rate to more adequate levels. (Refer to Table 5.3 for drug dosages.)

Asystole

Asystole is the complete absence of electrical activity of the heart in a nonbreathing, pulseless child. Usually the result of an unmanaged or mismanaged bradycardia secondary to hypoxia, asystole is a terminal rhythm. Similar to adults, children who present in asystole have poor outcomes with survival rates near 1%. Obviously the most effective intervention in aggressive airway management before the rhythm deteriorates. In cases where asystole is the presenting rhythm, airway management, effective CPR, and epinephrine are essential.

History

Obtaining a quick and accurate mechanism of injury, length of downtime, and any preexisting medical conditions are the only pieces of information required to begin intervention. This information should be obtained efficiently and in a nonaccusatory manner.

Assessment

The child in asystole will be unconscious, will have no spontaneous respirations, no pulse, and, therefore, no perfusion. The ECG will show a straight line. Occasional P waves may be noted and should not be interpreted as a perfusing rhythm (Figure 5.9A). Checking asystole in a perpendicular lead will confirm that it is not ventricular fibrillation or a problem with the monitor.

Management

BLS management includes the following steps:

- Initiate CPR.
- Control the airway and ventilate the child with a bag-valve mask.
- Keep the child warm.
- Provide rapid transport to the hospital.

ALS providers should additionally manage the child with the following:

- Intubate at once.
- Obtain IV or IO access.
- Consider possible causes of arrest:
  - hypoxia
  - hyperkalemia
  - hypokalemia
  - acidosis
  - drug overdose
  - hypothermia
- Attach a cardiac monitor and interpret the rhythm. If asystole is seen, continue CPR.
- Administer epinephrine and repeat it every 3 to 5 minutes. (Refer to Table 5.3 for recommended drug dosages and routes of administration.)
- Administer atropine every 3 to 5 minutes.
- Consider administration of other drugs according to local medical direction or protocols.

Ventricular Fibrillation

Ventricular fibrillation is the absence of any organized electrical activity in the heart, caused by multiple irritable foci in the myocardium randomly firing electrical impulses that are unable to initiate a mechanical contraction. It rarely occurs in children (only 10% of arrested patients), usually resulting from hypothermia, hypovolemia, electrocution, or drowning.

Defibrillation is the most desirable immediate therapy, but only when ventricular fibrillation is confirmed by ECG monitoring. Remember that most current automatic defibrillators are not approved for use in children.

History

Scene size-up may provide excellent clues about the mechanism of injury; however, a quick history is needed to determine downtime, any preexisting medical conditions, and care that has been provided by bystanders.

Assessment

The child with ventricular fibrillation will be unresponsive, pulseless, and apneic. The rhythm strip in ventricular fibrillation will show an irregular wave without identifiable P, QRS, or T waves. The height of the wave can classify the rhythm as either coarse or fine ventricular fibrillation, but this will not change the management in any way (Figure 5.9B).

Management

BLS management for ventricular fibrillation includes the following steps:

- Control the airway and ventilate with high-flow, high-concentration oxygen.
- Initiate CPR.
- Keep the child warm.
- Transport immediately to the hospital.

ALS providers should additionally manage the child with the following care:

- Intubate immediately.
- Obtain IV or IO access.
- Attach a cardiac monitor and interpret the rhythm. If ventricular fibrillation is seen, defibrillate as soon as possible at 2 J/kg (200 joules maximum) initially. If there is no success in establishing a

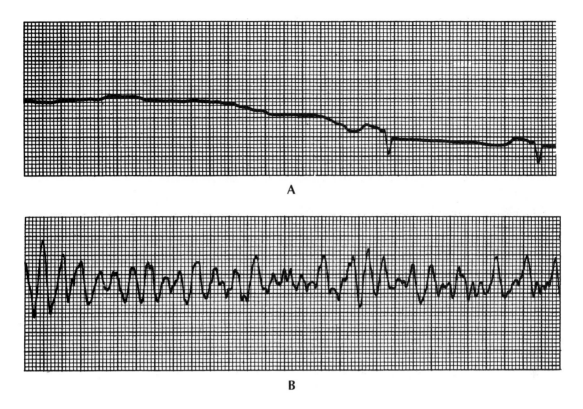

FIGURE 5.9 *(A) Asystole, (B) Ventricular fibrillation. (Reproduced with permission. Textbook of Pediatric Advanced Life Support, 1987. Copyright American Heart Association.)*

rhythm, double the energy does to 4 J/kg for second defibrillation. Defibrillation may be repeated once more at 4 J/kg if no rhythm is established. The time between shocks should be just long enough to check the rhythm.

- Administer epinephrine and repeat it every 3 to 5 minutes. (Refer to Table 5.3 for recommended drug dosages and routes of administration.)
- Repeat defibrillation at 4 J/kg within 30 to 60 seconds after each medication.
- Administer lidocaine every 3 to 5 minutes.
- Consider bretylium if the ventricular fibrillation is refractory to lidocaine.
- Consider other drugs according to local medical director or protocol.

Supraventricular Tachycardia

Supraventricular tachycardia is an episodic, serious dysrhythmia occurring in infants or older children, often near puberty. It is a rare but frightening disorder for parents and providers to treat, with an occurrence of 1 in 25,000 children. These children experience sustained heart rates in excess of 200/min, and often up to 300/min. It has been linked to prior cardiac surgery, but usually occurs in otherwise healthy children. There is no known trigger to the episode.

Children can sustain these heart rates for a while, but after several hours they may develop congestive heart failure. *It is a true medical emergency!*

TABLE 5.3A ■ *Drugs for Pediatric Resuscitation*

Drug Preparations Available	Dose/Route of Administration	Indication	Action	Adverse Effects
FIRST-LINE DRUGS				
Epinephrine				
1:10,000 Do not mix with sodium bicarbonate. 1:1000	0.01 mg/kg/dose IV, IO first dose for asystole and all doses for bradycardia 0.1 mg/kg/dose ET, subsequent doses IV or IO for asystole Repeat every 3–5 minutes.	Asystole, ventricular fibrillation, symptomatic bradycardia unresponsive to oxygen and ventilation	Alpha & beta adrenergic; increases heart rate, vasoconstriction, force of contraction, myocardial irritability; elevates blood pressure and coronary perfusion	Tachycardia Dysrhythmia Hypertension *Contraindicated* for irritable rhythms, ventricular tachycardia
Atropine				
0.1 mg/ml Do not mix with sodium bicarbonate.	0.02 mg/kg/dose IV, ET, or IO Minimum dose: 0.1 mg Maximum doses: single cumulative 0.5 mg 1.0 mg (children) 1.0 mg 2.0 mg (teens)	Bradycardia, but epinephrine is preferred. Increased vagal tone	Increases the heart rate	Tachycardia Dilated pupils *Contraindicated* for tachycardia, either sinus ventricular or atrial
Dextrose				
D50W Use D10W solution for neonates.	0.5–1.0 g/kg IV only Dilute D50W 1:1 with sterile water to D25W (2–4 ml/kg).	Unresponsive without mechanism, and no response to initial round of drugs, suspected hypoglycemia	Raises blood sugar level, needed for vigorous myocardia	Causes scarring of peripheral veins *Contraindicated* if known to be in diabetic ketoacidosis or blood glucose levels are normal
Narcan (Naloxone)				
0.4 mg/ml	0.1 mg/kg/dose initially Maximum dose: 0.8 mg IV push, may give ET If no response in 10 min, give 2 mg IV when narcotic overdose suspected.	Coma, respiratory depression, hypotension, known or suspected narcotic overdose	Antidote for narcotics	None listed
SECOND-LINE DRUGS				
Bretylium				
50 mg/ml	5 mg/kg/dose IV push Repeat q 15 min 10 mg/kg/dose to maximum dose 30 mg/kg	Ventricular dysrhythmias; lidocaine is not effective	Antiarrhythmic agent makes fibrillating heart susceptible to defibrillation.	Hypotension Bradyrhythmias Nausea, Vomiting Transient hypertension
Dopamine				
200 mg/5 ml Do not mix with sodium bicarbonate.	2–20 mcg/kg/min IV drip (6 mg × kg in 100 ml D5W) 1 ml/hr = 1 mcg/kg/min	Cardiogenic shock Hypotension Poor peripheral perfusion Stable rhythm	Renal vasodilation at low doses (2–5 mcg/kg), beta adrenergic effect, increases heart rate, cardiac contractility, and cardiac output	Tachycardia Dysrhythmia Hypertension *Contraindicated* in hypovolemic shock
Sodium Bicarbonate				
50 mEq/50 ml	First dose: 1 mEq/kg Second dose: 0.5 mgEq/kg IV push slowly Maximum dose: 3 mEq/kg Dilute 1:1 with D5W	Metabolic acidosis	Neutralizes acid pH, leads to CO_2 production	Metabolic alkalosis *Contraindicated* in cases of inadequate ventilation
Lidocaine				
10 mg/ml Concentration varies by drug company.	1.0 mg/kg/bolus dose IV or ET 15 minutes before beginning infusion Maximum dose of 50 mg IV 20–50 mcg/kg/min continuous drip	Recurrent ventricular tachycardia, ventricular fibrillation, or significant ventricular ectopy	Suppresses ventricular arrhythmias and ventricular ectopy	Hypotension Bradycardia Seizure Drowsiness Muscle twitching *Contraindicated* for asystole, heart block

TABLE 5.3B ■ *Drugs for Pediatric Disorders*

DRUG PREPARATIONS AVAILABLE	DOSE/ROUTE OF ADMINISTRATION	INDICATION	ACTION	ADVERSE EFFECTS
Valium (Diazepam)				
5 mg/ml Do not mix or dilute with other drugs or solutions.	0.2–0.3 mg/kg IV slow push over 3 min Inject as close to vein as possible. Maximum total dose: 5 mg ≤ 5 years old 10 mg ≥ 6 years old Repeat dose in 5–10 min if seizures continue.	Persistent seizure activity	Rapid action anticonvulsant	Respiratory depression; be prepared to assist ventilations.
Albuterol				
5 mg/ml	0.15 mg/kg initial dose Nebulizer, dilute in 2–3 ml saline 0.05 mg/kg every 20 min	Asthma	Bronchodilator, induces relaxation of bronchial smooth muscles	Tachycardia Vomiting
Epinephrine				
1:1000	0.01 mg/kg/dose Subcutaneous Maximum single dose 0.3 ml May be repeated every 20–30 min × 3 if heart rate is < 180	Asthma, expiratory respiratory distress, anaphylaxis	Rapid-action bronchodilator, induces relaxation of bronchial smooth muscle	Tachycardia Dysrhythmia Hypertension
Racemic Epinephrine				
2.25% solution	0.25–0.5 ml diluted in 2–3 ml Normal Saline, by nebulizer Dose/kg ratio: 0.25 ml if < 20 kg 0.5 ml if 20–40 kg	Croup, severe dyspnea, and a long transport time is anticipated.	May reduce respiratory distress	*Contraindicated* for marked tachycardia
Adenosine				
3 mg/ml	0.1–0.2 mg/kg IV push Maximum single dose: 12 mg	Supraventricular tachycardia	Produces transient heart block	Minimal because of short half-life

History

Important information to obtain during the history includes the following:

S Has the child's behavior changed to be more anxious or irritable? Has the child's level of responsiveness changed? Does the child feel faint or weak? Has the child experienced vomiting or other feeding problem?

A Does the child have any known allergies?

M Does the child take any medications? If so, for what health problem?

P Does the child have a heart defect? Has the child ever had heart surgery?

L What and when was the child's last oral intake?

E Has the child had any illness or injury lately? (This is different from shock from another cause.)

Assessment

Infants with supraventricular tachycardia will be pale or cyanotic, irritable, sweating, breathing rapidly, and feeding poorly or vomiting. They will have a regular heart rate too fast to count, about 240/min or higher. Signs of hypoperfusion (shock) may be present.

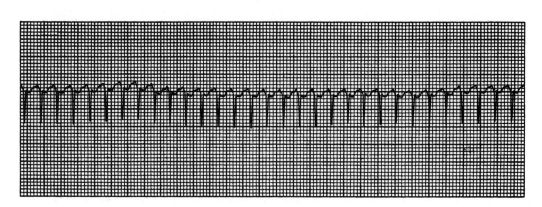

FIGURE 5.10 *Supraventricular tachycardia with a rate of 320 beats per minute. (Reproduced with permission.* Textbook of Pediatric Advanced Life Support, *1987. Copyright American Heart Association.)*

Older children will complain of feeling bad and have a fainting spell. Adolescents will have a regular heart rate between 150–250/min. Perfusion is poor so there will also be pallor or cyanosis and signs of shock. The child may recognize what is happening if this is a recurrent problem.

Supraventricular tachycardia will be exhibited by a rapid rate, no detectable variation in the R–R interval, lack of identifiable P waves, and narrow QRS complexes on rhythm strip (Figure 5.10).

Management

BLS field care for supraventricular tachycardia includes the following:

- Monitor ABCs and vital signs.
- Maintain airway control and administer high-flow, high-concentration oxygen by face mask.
- Prepare to administer CPR, and
- Transport immediately.
- Medical direction may recommend stimulation of the vagal nerve by placing an ice pack over the child's face.

ALS providers can provide the following additional care as medical direction or protocols direct:

- Attach a cardiac monitor and record a rhythm strip.
- Intubate the child if his or her level of responsiveness deteriorates. Ventilate with 100% oxygen before cardioversion unless hypoperfusion (shock) is present.
- Start an IV of Ringer's Lactate or Normal Saline at a keep-open rate.
- Perform cardioversion at 0.5 J/kg, using pediatric paddles (minimal setting on some defibrillators is 5J). If the attempt is unsuccessful, repeat doubling the energy charge.
- Give medications according to local protocols if an IV is in place.

Guidelines for Drug Administration

There are four first-line drugs used during the resuscitation of children. There are also some additional drugs used for specific circumstances (Table 5.3).

The intravenous route is preferred for drug administration during a cardiac arrest; however, establishing a peripheral line is not easily accomplished in children, particularly those in shock. The endotracheal tube and intraosseous site are alternate routes for drug administration. Often prehospital providers are directed to obtain an IV line during transport rather than delay transport for this procedure.

It is currently recommended that the drug dosage used for endotracheal administration be double or triple the IV dose, except epinephrine, which should be given at 10 times the IV dose. Unless special care is taken when giving small doses of the drugs through the endotracheal tube, some of the drug remains on the tube, never making contact with the lung tissue for absorption. Drugs administered to children through the endotracheal tube should be diluted in 3–5 cc of Normal Saline. The drug should then be injected into the endotracheal tube as deeply as possible, using a 6–8 French feeding tube or suction catheter. This is followed by several positive pressure ventilations. The drug may alternately be injected into the endotracheal tube, which is then flushed with 2–3 ml of Normal Saline.

Drug absorption from the bone marrow is considered as good as an IV injection. When administering drugs by either of these routes, it is important to flush the IV line with 5 ml of saline to make sure all of the drug is delivered and that drug interactions are avoided.

Some drugs are given by nebulizer so that liquid medications are transformed into aerosol (water particles in which the drug is dissolved or suspended) to work by direct contact with the airway and lung tissues. The medication should be place in the "aerosol kit" cup with enough saline to equal 3 ml. The tubing should then be connected to the oxygen flow meter, set at 10 l/min. The medication is then given to the child, using a mouthpiece, mask, or blow-by method, whichever best suits the child's age, mental status, and level of cooperation.

Pediatric CPR References

Accident Facts: 1995 Edition. Itasca, IL: National Safety Council, 1995.

Chameides, L., "CPR challenges in pediatrics," *Annals of Emergency Medicine,* 22, no. 2 (1993), pp. 281–288.

Chameides, L., and Hazinski, M.F., eds., *Textbook of Pediatric Advanced Life Support,* 2nd ed. Dallas: American Heart Association, 1994.

Children's National Medical Center Formulary: Pediatric Drug Therapy and Formulary Handbook. Hudson, OH: Lexicomp, 1995.

Coffin, C.R., Quan, L., Graves, J.R., et al., "Etiologies and outcomes of the pulseless, nonbreathing pediatric patient presenting with ventricular fibrillation," *Annals of Emergency Medicine,* 21, no. 9 (September 1992), p. 1046.

Eisenberg, M., Bergner, L., and Hallstrom, A., "Epidemiology of cardiac arrest and resuscitation in children," *Annals of Emergency Medicine,* 12, no. 11 (November 1983), pp. 672–674.

Emergency Cardiac Core Committee and Subcommittees, American Heart Association, "Guidelines for cardiopulmonary resuscitation and emergency cardiac care, VI: Pediatric advanced life support," *JAMA,* 268, no. 16 (October 28, 1992), pp. 2262–2275.

_____. "Guidelines for cardiopulmonary resuscitation and emergency cardiac care, V: Pediatric basic life support," *JAMA,* 268, no. 16 (October 28, 1992), pp. 2251–2261.

_____. "Guidelines for cardiopulmonary resuscitation and emergency cardiac care, IX: Ensuring effectiveness of community wide emergency cardiac care," *JAMA,* 268, no. 16 (October 28, 1992), pp. 2289–2295.

Goetting, M.G., "Progress in pediatric cardiopulmonary resuscitation," *Emergency Clinics of North America,* 13, no. 2 (May 1995), pp. 291–319.

Harris, C.S., et al., "Childhood asphyxiation by food," *JAMA, 251,* no. 17 (1984), pp. 2231–2235.

Jones, S., and Bagg, A.M., "Lead drugs for cardiac arrest," *Nursing,* 88, 18, no. 1 (January 1988), pp. 34–42.

Losek, J.D., et al., "Prehospital care of the pulseless, nonbreathing pediatric patient," *American Journal of Emergency Medicine,* 5, no. 5 (May 1987), pp. 370–374.

Nichols, D.G., Yaster, M., Lappe, D.G., and Buck, J.R., *Golden Hour: The Handbook of Advanced Pediatric Life Support.* St. Louis: Mosby Year Book, Inc., 1991.

Reynolds, L.M., Nicolson, S.C., Seven, J.M., McGonigle, M.E., and Jobes, D.R., "Influence of sensor site location on pulse oximetry kinetics in children," *Anesthesia Analgesia,* 76, no. 3 (1993), pp. 751–754.

Schoenfeld, P.S., and Baker, M.D., "Management of cardiopulmonary and trauma resuscitation in the pediatric emergency department," *Pediatrics,* 91, no. 4 (April 1993), pp. 726–729.

Seidel, J.S., and Henderson, D.P., eds., *Prehospital Care of Pediatric Emergencies.* Los Angeles: Pediatric Society of California, 1987.

Silverman, B.J., ed., *Advanced Pediatric Life Support.* Dallas: American College of Emergency Physicians, 1994.

Tendrup, T.E., Kanter, R.K., and Cherry, R.A., "A comparison of infant ventilation methods performed by prehospital personnel," *Annals of Emergency Medicine,* 18, no. 6 (1989), pp. 607–611.

Respiratory Emergencies

OBJECTIVES

When you have completed this chapter you should be able to

▶ List the five most common respiratory emergencies in children.
▶ Describe the findings that differentiate between various upper and lower airway emergencies.
▶ Describe the management of acute respiratory distress in the child with asthma, bronchiolitis, croup, or epiglottitis.
▶ Describe the management of drowning and near-drowning.

Introduction

Because of their association with acute respiratory distress and hypoxia, conditions involving the respiratory tract should immediately alert you to be especially vigilant in assessing the child, monitoring the respiratory rate, and evaluating the progression of symptoms.

Children have lower resistance to viruses and bacteria; consequently, infants and small children are at greater risk of respiratory infections. The small diameter of their airway is susceptible to obstruction from foreign bodies and swelling. In addition, the smooth muscle in their airway is more reactive to pollutants and foreign bodies, also resulting in acute respiratory distress.

The most common respiratory disorders you will treat in the prehospital setting include croup, epiglottitis, asthma, bronchiolitis, and foreign-body aspiration. See Chapter 5 "Pediatric Cardiopulmonary Resuscitation," for information on foreign-body obstruction of the airway.

Asthma

Asthma is a chronic recurrent lower airway disease producing moderate to severe respiratory distress. The most common age of onset is the preschool years, but it may be diagnosed in children as young as 1 year of age. It is the most serious allergic disease in children and a leading cause of missed school days. The mortality rate has risen for the past two decades.

The obstruction of the lower airways is caused by a sensitivity reaction to foods, inhalants, pollens, mold spores, or a combination of these allergens. Other factors contributing to the episodes of asthma include changes in temperature, physical exertion, psychologic stress, and respiratory infections.

The allergic response produces edema, increased secretion of thick mucus from the bronchial glands, and spasm of the bronchioles and bronchi (Figure 6.1). The mucus, bronchial spasm, and edema decrease the size of the bronchioles, causing a lower airway obstruction. The child develops respiratory distress and hypoxia. The expiratory phase of breathing becomes prolonged and forceful with noticeable wheezing as the child attempts to expire air beyond the obstructions. Dehydration of the airway, caused by breathing through the mouth, increases the thickness of the mucus and respiratory distress.

History

Important information to obtain during the history includes the following:

S   Is the child experiencing trouble breathing? Are accessory muscles being used? Are wheezes or other noises easily heard?

A   Does the child have any allergies or allergic condition?

M   Does the child take any medications? Any medications for asthma, either oral or inhalant? Have any medications been used for this attack? Did the medications relieve any of the symptoms?

P   Has the child ever had an asthma attack? Has anyone in the family ever had asthma or other allergic condition? Has the child ever been admitted to an intensive care unit for an asthma attack?

L   How much liquid has the child been drinking?

E   Does the child have any other illnesses or fever? Has it been treated?

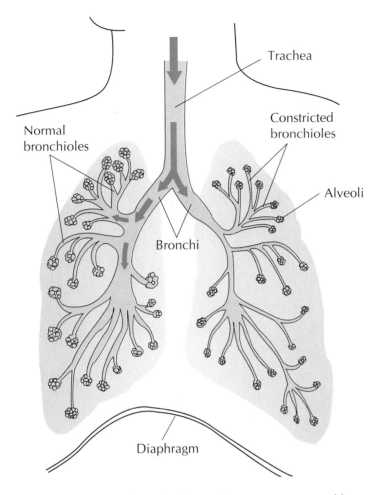

Trachea

Constricted
bronchioles

Normal
bronchioles

Alveoli

Bronchi

Diaphragm

FIGURE 6.1 *In asthma the lower airways are narrowed by
constriction of bronchiole muscles and secretion of thick
mucus, causing a lower airway obstruction.*

Assessment

The child with an acute asthma attack is in respiratory distress with
shortness of breath, tachypnea, tachycardia, noticeable expiratory wheezing, intercostal retractions, and nasal flaring. The child has coughing
episodes, attempting to clear the obstructing mucus. These episodes often
trigger vomiting.

The patient often appears pale or mottled. The lips may be a deep,
dark red color that progresses to cyanosis as the hypoxia increases. The
child is generally apprehensive and restless, and mental status may further deteriorate if hypoxia is not controlled. The young child may be most
comfortable in the tripod position. Older children might brace themselves
over a chair to facilitate the use of accessory muscles (Figure 6.2). Breath
sounds are usually bilateral with coarse rhonchi and generalized inspiratory and expiratory wheezing.

Breath sounds may diminish, indicating progression of the obstruction and little movement of air. Expiration is prolonged as the child
attempts to move inspired air beyond the obstruction. Shallow or irregular respirations, or a decrease in respiratory rate, are serious signs of
imminent ventilatory failure.

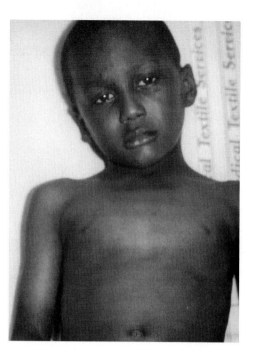

FIGURE 6.2 *Child in respiratory distress from asthma.*

Management

BLS field care for asthma includes the following:

- Assess and monitor ABCDEs.
- Administer high-flow, high-concentration oxygen by face mask. Humidified oxygen will help loosen lower airway secretions, further opening the bronchioles.
- Maintain the child's airway and be alert to the possibility of vomiting and need for suctioning.
- If the child has an inhaler or bronchodilator, assist the parent or child in administering it.
- If the child's mental status is intact, and there is no fear of aspiration, encourage him or her to drink some water or clear liquid while en route to the hospital.
- Be prepared for ventilatory failure. Administer positive pressure ventilation and CPR if indicated.
- Transport patient immediately. Let the child determine position of comfort during transport.

ALS personnel may want to provide additional treatment as directed by medical direction or protocol:

- Administer a beta agonist, such as albuterol, according to local protocols.
- Start an IV with Ringer's Lactate or Normal Saline at a keep-open rate.
- Endotracheal intubation should be performed if airway management becomes difficult or ventilatory failure occurs.

Status Asthmaticus

Children who continue with acute signs of respiratory distress despite treatment are considered to be in *status asthmaticus.* The child can move only a small amount of air. So little air is moved that wheezing may not be heard. The patient is cyanotic, pulse rate is elevated, and breathing obviously is labored. Humidified oxygen is required and intubation should be considered. Transport to the hospital is needed immediately.

Bronchiolitis

Bronchiolitis is an infection of the lower respiratory tract, most often caused by the respiratory syncytial virus (RSV), or parainfluenza virus. The illness usually begins with a mild fever, runny nose, and cough that gradually progresses to respiratory distress. The bronchioles in the lower airway become obstructed with edema and increased mucous secretion due to the inflammatory process of the viral illness. It most often affects infants between 2 months and 18 months of age and may recur. Recurrence may be associated with a different viral infection in the infant with a sensitive airway.

History

Important information to obtain during the history includes the following:

S   What symptoms does the infant have and how have they changed over time? When did symptoms become this severe?
A   Does the child have any allergies?
M   What medications or treatments have been given?
P   Has the child ever had any symptoms like this before?
L   How much liquid has the child been drinking?
E   Has the child had any fever and has it been treated?

Assessment

When you arrive at the scene, the infant is in acute respiratory distress with difficulty breathing and irritability. In the older infant, it is difficult to distinguish between bronchiolitis and asthma.

The child may have a mild fever and a dry cough. Nasal flaring, tachypnea, tachycardia, and intercostal and suprasternal retractions will all be present. Inspiratory and expiratory wheezing is heard bilaterally when auscultating the chest. The infant will be restless and anxious when respiratory distress is severe. Mild dehydration may be present, lasting a few days, as a result of the fever and the generalized illness.

Management

BLS field care for bronchiolitis includes the following:

- Assess and monitor ABCDEs.
- Clear nasal passages and maintain airway.
- Administer high-flow, high-concentration oxygen by face mask. Use humidified oxygen if available.
- Be prepared for ventilatory failure. Administer positive pressure ventilation and CPR if indicated.
- Transport the patient immediately. Allow the child to select his or her own position of comfort.

ALS personnel may want to provide additional treatment as directed by medical direction or protocol.

- Start an IV of Ringer's Lactate or Normal Saline at a keep-open rate.
- Consider a beta agonist, such as albuterol, and administer according to medical direction or local protocols.
- Nebulized sterile water may also be beneficial.

Croup

Croup, a viral upper respiratory infection, commonly occurs in children between 6 months and 3 years of age. The infection localizes in the upper airway, leading to swelling of the larynx and subglottic tissue, and occasionally the trachea and bronchi (Figure 6.3A). The child usually has cold symptoms (runny nose, nasal congestion, sneezing, and mild fever) with an onset over 1 to 3 days. The child then develops the characteristic barking (seal-like) cough. The disorder tends to occur more commonly in the spring and fall and may recur in the same child.

History

Important information to obtain during the history includes the following:

S   What symptoms does the child have (fever, cough, runny nose, sore throat, etc.)? Have these symptoms changed over the last few hours? Does the child have any difficulties swallowing liquids? Is he or she drooling saliva?
A   Does the child have any allergies?
M   What medications has the child been given?
P   How long has the child been ill? Has the child recently been to the doctor for this problem? Has the patient ever had symptoms like this before?
L   How much liquid has the child been drinking?
E   What other treatment has been tried at home (vaporizer, steam in bathroom, exposure to cold night air)? How effective was the treatment?

Assessment

In most cases you will be summoned for a child in moderate to severe respiratory distress. The onset is usually gradual and symptoms may have been present for several days. Signs and symptoms of the child with croup include the following:

- Signs of respiratory distress, such as nasal flaring, tachypnea, retractions (intercostal, supracostal, and sternal in severe cases), tachycardia, tachypnea, and pallor or cyanosis.
- The characteristic seal-like barking cough that worsens as the airway obstruction increases.
- Hoarse cry or hoarse voice.
- Inspiratory stridor and expiratory stridor in severe cases.
- Anxious, restless, noticeable decrease in activity level.
- Altered level of responsiveness in severe cases.
- A low-grade fever may be present.

On physical examination the infant or child appears anxious and in respiratory distress. Breath sounds may be decreased in severe distress.

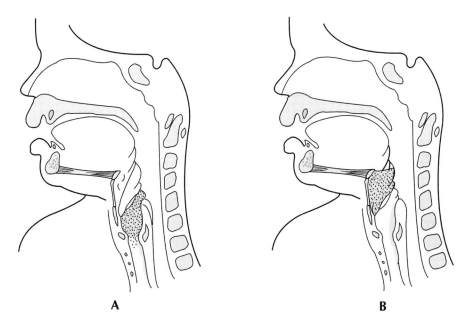

FIGURE 6.3 (A) Croup; note swelling of the larynx and subglottic tissue in contrast to (B) epiglottitis with swelling of and above the epiglottis.

In less severe cases, you may hear expiratory and inspiratory wheezing, or harsh rhonchi. Use Table 6.1 to assess and describe the severity of croup to medical direction.

In the prehospital setting, the croup score is generally not calculated. Rather, it is important to assess each of the individual signs for severity.

TABLE 6.1 ■ *Croup Scale to Identify the Severity of Croup*

	SEVERITY SCORE			
SIGNS	0	1	2	3
Stridor	None	Mild	Moderate at rest	Severe, on the inspiration + expiration
Retractions	None	Mild	Suprasternal, intercostal	Severe, may see sternal retractions
Color	Normal	Normal score = 0	Normal score = 0	Dusky or cyanotic
Breath Sounds	Normal	Mildly decreased	Moderately decreased	Markedly decreased
Level of Responsiveness	Normal	Restless when disturbed	Anxious, agitated	Lethargic

SCORING: To quantify the severity of croup, add up the individual scores for each of the sign categories. A score between 0 to 15 is possible. The rating of mild, moderate, and severe is as follows:

    4–5 is mild.
    6–8 is moderate.
    > 8 or any sign in the severe category is severe.

Source: Adapted from Davis, H.W., et al., (1981): "Acute upper airway obstruction, croup, and epiglottitis," *Pediatric Clinics of North America,* 28:4.

Medical direction will be most interested in the specific findings noted with each sign rather than the total score. Croup is considered severe any time a child has even one sign among the severe findings on this croup scale, which include the following:

- Lethargy, altered level of responsiveness;
- Severe stridor, on inspiration and expiration;
- Severe retractions, which may include sternal retractions;
- Dusky or cyanotic color; and
- Markedly decreased breath sounds.

Management

BLS field care for croup is the same as for any respiratory distress.

- Monitor ABCDEs and vital signs.
- Administer high-flow, high concentration oxygen by face mask if the child will tolerate it, or administer blow-by oxygen.
- If the child is awake and conscious, do not agitate the child with excessive physical examination or handling.
- Do not attempt to visualize the mouth and throat or use instruments in the airway, since it is often difficult to distinguish between croup and epiglottitis in the prehospital setting.
- In cases of sever respiratory distress, be prepared for respiratory arrest; implement positive pressure ventilation and CPR as necessary.
- Transport patient and contact medical direction. Let the child choose the position of comfort for transport, either sitting up or lying down.

ALS providers may want to provide the following care, according to protocol or medical direction.

- Start an IV of Ringer's Lactate or Normal Saline at a keep-open rate or as ordered by medical direction.
- Racemic epinephrine by positive pressure ventilation.

Epiglottitis

Epiglottitis is a bacterial infection localized in the epiglottis, usually caused by *Hemophilus influenzae*, type B. Acute swelling occurs above the glottis, creating an airway obstruction (Figure 6.3B). It most commonly affects children between 3 to 6 years of age; however, it does occur in young infants, older children, and adults. Because of the sudden onset and rapid progression of respiratory distress and airway obstruction, the child with epiglottitis is a true medical emergency. Often the child will awaken with a sudden-onset high fever, difficulty breathing, sore throat, and difficulty swallowing.

History

Important information to obtain during the history includes the following:

S   Does the child have a sore throat? Will the child drink and swallow liquids or saliva? Is the child drooling? Is the child's voice hoarse or muffled?
A   Does the child have any allergies?

M   Has the child been given any medications?

P   Does the child have a fever? How high is the fever? Has the child ever had an illness like this before?

L   How much liquid has the child been able to drink?

E   When did the child first become ill? Is this a recent illness with sudden worsening, or is this an illness with sudden onset?

Assessment

When you arrive at the scene, the child with epiglottitis will appear sick, have a high fever (up to 102°–103°F), and experience difficulty breathing. The patient is in acute distress with a severe airway obstruction and may be in a tripod position, in which the child sits upright with his or her neck extended forward and the weight of the body resting on the patient's outstretched arms in front (Figure 6.4). This position maximizes the airway opening around the swollen epiglottis.

The child generally holds the mouth open with the tongue protruding slightly, almost like holding a piece of hot potato on the tongue. The pain from the sore throat is intense, resulting in the refusal to swallow saliva or other liquids. This child looks anxious and is very focused on each slow, deliberate breath. The child will be lethargic and show very little concern for what is happening around him or her (Figure 6.5).

The child will be experiencing hypoxia and respiratory distress. Typical signs of respiratory distress, such as nasal flaring and intercostal and suprasternal retractions, will be present. Occasionally a muffled voice or stridor will be present; however, there is rarely a cough. Respiratory rate will generally not be increased. The child will have tachycardia and cyanosis in cases of progressive hypoxia.

The child with epiglottitis should be identified immediately from initial observation and history of the patient. Do not attempt to examine the child's mouth.

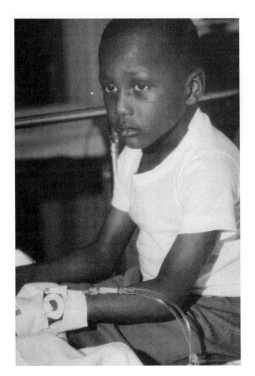

FIGURE 6.4   *Child sitting in tripod position.*

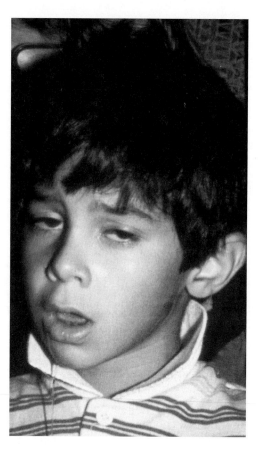

FIGURE 6.5 *Classic appearance of child with epiglottitis. (From* Atlas of Pediatric Physical Diagnosis *by Davis Zitelli, 1987, Mosby International, London, UK. Reprinted with permission.)*

Management

BLS field care for the child with suspected epiglottitis includes the following:

- Monitor ABCDEs and vital signs.
- *DO NOT* MANIPULATE THE AIRWAY IN ANY WAY! *DO NOT* attempt to visualize, insert a tongue blade, or shine a flashlight into the patient's mouth. It may produce a laryngospasm and totally occlude the airway.
- Permit the child to remain sitting. *DO NOT* attempt to have the child lie down; the swollen epiglottis can fall back into the airway and cause obstruction.
- Minimize handling and examining of the child to prevent agitation and crying.
- Keep child with the parent or primary caretaker at all times.
- Administer high-flow, high-concentration oxygen by face mask. Approach the child very gently with the oxygen mask or give the mask to the parent to hold. If the mask distresses the child, administer oxygen via blow-by.
- Transport immediately. Notify the hospital to be prepared for a child with suspected epiglottitis.
- If an airway obstruction occurs, administer positive pressure ventilation with high-concentration, high-flow oxygen after getting a good seal. Use enough pressure to get beyond the obstruction; however, be prepared for gastric distention. Some oxygen will get beyond the obstruction and buy time until you get the child to the hospital.
- Perform CPR as indicated.

ALS providers will not need to provide any additional care beyond that of BLS providers. Field intubation of the child with epiglottitis is contraindicated. The swollen epiglottis totally obliterates the larynx and other landmarks used for tube insertion. In addition, the manipulation of the mouth and throat with the laryngoscope may trigger a total airway obstruction.

Intubation for epiglottitis is performed by the most skilled physician or anesthesiologist in a controlled setting of the hospital, usually the operating room. An emergency tracheostomy can then be performed if intubation is not successful. If the child experiences a total airway obstruction en route to the hospital, and positive pressure ventilation is not effective, medical direction may order a cricothyrotomy to establish an airway. While this procedure may be life-saving, it is difficult to perform in the young child.

Drowning and Near-Drowning

Drowning is defined as death within 24 hours following a submersion in a liquid medium. *Near-drowning* describes a submersion incident in which the child survives at least 24 hours, but death may ultimately occur. Drowning is a leading cause of preventable death to children in the United States, accounting for nearly 1600 deaths to children under 20 years of age in 1991.

Among young children the majority of drowning episodes occur when there is a short lapse in supervision, lasting only a few minutes. These episodes usually occur in fresh water (pools, lakes, bathtubs, buckets, toilets, and fish tanks). Children under 3 years of age are helpless in water, and because they are top-heavy, often cannot extricate and save themselves when falling head first into buckets, bathtubs, pools, etc. Drowning incidents in older children and adolescents are often related to boating errors, exhaustion after attempting to swim long distances, and alcohol use. Children with seizures are four times more like to drown if permitted to swim unsupervised.

The child who is trapped in water panics and struggles, initially holding his or her breath. Then the child swallows water, vomits, and cannot avoid aspirating water and vomitus. Some children develop laryngospasm, and if it persists beyond loss of consciousness and cessation of respiratory effort, there is no aspiration of water (dry drowning). Up to 80% of all drowning events will be "wet" drowning events with water and vomitus in the lungs.

During the submersion, the child develops hypoxia, acidosis, and cardiac arrest, leading to initial brain damage. Factors associated with the child's outcome after submersion include the following:

- Total submersion time,
- How quickly the resuscitation efforts began following rescue, and
- The temperature of the water.

The child who drowns in cold water becomes hypothermic very quickly because of the large body surface area to mass ratio. This reduces the metabolic rate and demand for oxygen, resulting in bradycardia. A protective mechanism preferentially shunts blood to the brain and heart. Rapid cooling may partially protect children from significant brain damage. Children have been successfully resuscitated after submersion in cold water for up to one hour.

History

Important information to obtain at the time of rescue includes the following:

S Did the child have any spontaneous respiratory effort upon rescue? Was there a heart rate?

A

M

P Does the child have seizures, diabetes, or another medical condition?

L

E How long was the child submerged? How quickly did resuscitation begin following rescue? What is the approximate water temperature? Was the child diving in shallow water?

Assessment

During the initial assessment, note the presence of any spontaneous respiratory effort and a heart rate, even if very slow. Spontaneous respirations are an indicator of full recovery. In most cases, the child will be unresponsive, pulseless, and have no spontaneous respiratory effort.

Management

BLS management for drowning and near-drowning victims includes the following:

- Scene size-up.
- Assess ABCs and vital signs.
- Control the airway and protect the C-spine, especially if trauma is suspected.
- Clear the airway if obstructed.
- Begin assisted ventilations with high-flow, high-concentration oxygen if no spontaneous breathing is apparent (Figure 6.6).

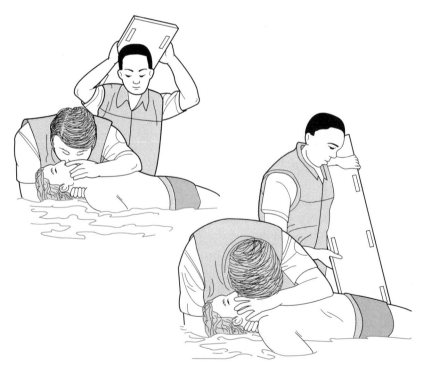

FIGURE 6.6 *Begin rescue breathing to the drowning victim as soon as you have access to the child.*

- Begin CPR if no heart rate is palpable.
- Remove wet clothing and wrap victim in blankets.
- If hypothermic, wrap in dry blankets and initiate rewarming measures while en route. Place heat packs along the torso of the body, protecting the skin from burns (if local guidelines permit). Follow BLS care guidelines in Chapter 7.
- Transport patient immediately to a hospital capable of providing pediatric intensive care, when available.

ALS providers should additionally initiate the following care:

- Intubate the child if there is no respiratory effort.
- Assess breath sounds and consider deep endotracheal suctioning.
- Establish an IV line with Ringer's Lactate or Normal Saline (warmed if available) at a keep-open rate. An IO line may be used for children under 6 years of age requiring medications and fluids.
- Initiate the PALS (Pediatric Advanced Life Support) drug protocol if the child is not hypothermic. (See dosages on Table 5.3.)

CAUTION!

DROWNING WITH SEVERE HYPOTHERMIA

If a heart rate is present, even if very slow, no invasive management should be attempted, including chest compressions. Such a maneuver may irritate the vagus nerve, resulting in asystole. With severe bradycardia, some perfusion of the brain is occurring, and the hypothermia stimulates the body to shunt blood only to the major organs. In this case, it would be better to assist ventilations with high-flow, high-concentration oxygen during transport.

Respiratory Emergency References

Bank, D.E., and Krug, S.E., "New approaches to upper airway disease," *Emergency Medical Clinics of North America*, 13, no. 2 (May 1995), pp. 473–487.

Barkin, R.M., "Pediatric respiratory emergencies," *Emergency Care Quarterly*, 5, no. 1 (May 1989), pp. 71–78.

Bledsoe, B.E., "Pediatric respiratory emergencies," *JEMS*, 19, no. 2 (February 1994), pp. 38–49.

Chameides, L., and Hazinski, M.F., eds., *Textbook of Pediatric Advanced Life Support*, 2nd ed., Dallas: American Heart Association, 1994.

Children's National Medical Center Formulary: Pediatric Drug Therapy and Formulary Handbook. Hudson, OH: Lexicomp, 1995.

Clark, J.R., "The perils of puddles, pails, and pools: Preparing for pediatric submersions," *JEMS*, 17, no. 6 (June 1992), pp. 38–44.

Cohen, H.C., "Attacking asthma in the prehospital setting," *JEMS*, 16, no. 8 (August 1991), pp. 81–92.

Fletcher, H.J., Ibrahim, S.A., and Speight, N., "Survey of asthma deaths in the northern region 1970–1985," *Archives of Disease in Childhood*, 65, no. 2 (February 1990), p. 163.

Matera, P., "Breathe easy: Diagnosing and treating asthma in the field," *JEMS*, 18, no. 11 (November 1993), pp. 40–51.

Werdmann, M.J., "Pediatric drowning," *Emergency*, 26, no. 8 (August 1994), pp. 28–33.

7

Medical Emergencies

OBJECTIVES

When you have completed this chapter you should be able to

▶ Describe fever and hypothermia, identifying their impact on managing the child with other emergencies.

▶ Describe field management for the child with a seizure.

▶ Describe field management for meningitis and sepsis, including special precautions for both patient and prehospital provider.

▶ Differentiate among mild, moderate, and severe dehydration.

▶ Describe the physical signs and prehospital management for diabetic ketoacidosis (hyperglycemia) and hypoglycemia.

▶ Describe care for the child in anaphylactic shock.

▶ List signs of distress in a child with a congenital heart defect.

▶ Describe the appropriate prehospital care of children at home with high-technology equipment.

Hyperthermia: Fever

Fever is defined as a core body temperature over 100.5°F or 38°C. A temperature of 101°F (38.4°C) or higher is generally cause for concern. Fever usually results from the body's response to an acute viral or bacterial infection. Bacteria or viruses cause the body's thermostat to set at a higher level, and the body responds by generating and retaining body heat. It is believed that fever is a protective response enabling the body to mobilize and fight the infection.

Fever or hyperthermia may also result from an alteration in the brain's ability to regulate body temperature. Various drugs in toxic doses (aspirin, atropine, and antihistamines) can cause hyperthermia by altering the brain's regulation of temperature. Children frequently have a febrile response to illnesses, with a range of temperature between 101° and 105°F. Higher temperatures may be present, but *neurologic damage does not occur until the temperature reaches 107°F.*

Fever from an acute illness is generally not a significant prehospital problem unless the child has a febrile seizure. *Febrile seizures* are most common in children under 5 years of age. A febrile seizure is most often triggered by the rapid rise in temperature, rather than the ultimate high temperature. If you find a child at the scene with a 105°F temperature who has not yet had a febrile seizure, it is unlikely that the child will convulse or have a seizure.

Hyperthermia may also result from exposure during hot weather. The child has less ability to reduce body temperature than to produce heat and raise body temperature. Situations producing hyperthermia are sitting in a closed car or an apartment during hot weather, which results in either heat exhaustion or heat stroke. The child's core temperature will rapidly rise to dangerous temperature levels, greater than 106°F. This rapid rise in core body temperature is associated with an increased oxygen demand and metabolic acidosis. This seriously strains the cardiac and respiratory systems, leading to respiratory and ventilatory failure.

History

Important information to obtain during the history includes the following:

S   What symptoms are present with the fever, such as trouble breathing, vomiting, diarrhea, change in behavior or level of responsiveness? Has the child had a seizure? Does the parent or caretaker know the child's temperature? How long ago was the temperature taken?

A   Does the child have any known allergies?

M   Have any medications been given for the fever such as aspirin, acetaminophen, or ibuprofen? How long ago? What was the response to the medication? Does the child take any other medications?

P   Does the child have any chronic illnesses or other health problems? Has the child been seen by a physician or other health professional for this illness? What health problem was identified?

L   What did the child last have to eat or drink? How long ago?

E   Where was the child found? What was the temperature of the environment?

Assessment

During the initial assessment and detailed physical exam, look for signs and symptoms associated with a fever. These include the following:

- Flushed, warm/hot skin;
- Chills and shivering (in some cases); complaints of feeling cold;
- Increased perspiration (less common in infants);
- Tachycardia and tachypnea (for each degree of temperature rise, the heart rate increases 8 to 10 beats per minute, and the respiratory rate increases 2 to 3 breaths per minute);
- Malaise, vague aches and pains;
- Signs of dehydration, dry mucous membranes;
- Decreased responsiveness (listless, lethargic, or irritable); and
- Loss of appetite.

In cases of heat stroke, the child may rapidly progress from severe headache to fainting, stiff neck, coma, posturing, and seizures, in addition to the above signs of a fever. Sweating may or may not be present.

The degree of temperature elevation is not necessarily associated with the seriousness of the patient's illness. Observe the child's response to the fever to determine the seriousness of the illness. You should be more concerned with a lethargic child having a 102°F temperature than the child who is alert and playful with a 105°F temperature.

You should also be more concerned if the febrile child has a chronic illness such as a congenital heart defect, leukemia or cancer, HIV infection or AIDs, sickle cell disease, or hydrocephalus controlled with a shunt. These children may have a very serious infection requiring urgent medical care.

Management

BLS care for a febrile infant or child should include the following:

- Monitor ABCs and vital signs. If a thermometer or skin temperature strip is available, obtain a temperature reading.
- Remove heavy clothing.
- Give oral liquids if the child is alert, able to swallow, and not vomiting or having diarrhea (usually not recommended for short transport times).
- Prepare for a possible seizure.
- In cases of exposure hyperthermia, administer high-flow, high-concentration oxygen by face mask and prepare to assist ventilations. For each degree of temperature rise, there is a 12% increase in oxygen consumption.
- Begin rapid cooling by removing patient's clothes, placing patient in a cool environment, and begin sponging.
- Transport patient rapidly in cases of exposure hyperthermia. In cases of acute, non-life-threatening illness, encourage the parent to take the child with a fever to the family physician (if local protocols or medical direction permit).

ALS providers may additionally want to provide the following care:

- Start an IV with Ringer's Lactate or Normal Saline at a keep-open rate. Fluid replacement may be needed by some children.
- Endotracheal intubation if the child's level of responsiveness begins to deteriorate.

CAUTION!

Hypothermia

Hypothermia is a core body temperature of less than 95°F (35°C). In children it most often results from prolonged exposure to cold temperatures. Children have a proportionately larger body surface area for their weight than do adults. Their temperature regulation mechanism is also less well developed, so their heat conservation efforts are less effective. Newborns have even greater risk of hypothermia because they have little subcutaneous fat. Causes of hypothermia include:

- Exposure to cool and cold weather;
- Ingestion of alcohol and drugs such as barbiturates (they dilate the peripheral blood vessels and interfere with the body's ability to conserve heat);
- Metabolic problems such as hypoglycemia;
- Trauma or other brain disorders that interfere with the temperature-regulating system; and
- Overwhelming infection (sepsis).

Heat loss is accelerated by wet clothes and high winds through the process of convection and conduction. Submersion in cold water has the most profound effect on heat loss and is further intensified by any movement. Death can occur in as short a time as 15 minutes. If the diving reflex is triggered during rapid cooling, a young child may be successfully resuscitated after a longer period of time. (See "Drowning and Near-Drowning" in Chapter 6.)

The progressive response of the body to lowered core body temperatures is as follows:

- The brain senses blood cooling in the extremities and triggers increased muscle tone and a higher metabolic rate.
- Shivering begins when muscle tone is increased.
- Constriction of blood vessels leads to pooling of cool blood in the extremities.

The body is able to increase heat production at about 4 times its normal rate with these efforts. The core body temperature begins to drop when these functions can no longer compensate for the environmental cold.

History

Important information to obtain during the history includes the following:

S Is the child shivering? Is the child's level of responsiveness decreased or is the child unconscious? Is the skin surface cool or cold to the touch? Is the skin color pale, mottled, or cyanotic? Does the child have sensation in skin surfaces exposed to the environment?

A Does the child have any known allergies?

M Does the child take any medications? Were any drugs or alcohol ingested that could interfere with body temperature regulation?

P Does the child have any chronic illnesses or other health problems?

L When was the child's last oral intake? What was it?

E How long has the child been exposed to the cold environment? What is the estimated temperature? Was the cold exposure associated with water, such as soaking with rain or submersion in cold water?

Assessment

The child will present with progressively deteriorating signs and symptoms as the core body temperature drops (Table 7.1). Prolonged vasoconstriction is accompanied by a decrease in tissue temperatures and may result in local cold injury or frostbite.

Thickening of the blood may lead to clotting, and ice crystals may form when the tissue temperature nears 0°C. The ears, nose, fingers, toes, hands, and feet are most often affected by frostbite. A superficial injury is indicated by pain and flushed, burning skin. A deeper injury is indicated by blistering and loss of sensation.

Management

BLS care for mild hypothermia includes the following (Figure 7.1):

■ Move patient to warm environment.
■ Remove wet clothing and wrap patient in blankets to passively rewarm.
■ Give warm liquids by mouth if the child is conscious.

BLS field care for moderate to severe hypothermia includes the following steps:

■ Maintain the airway.
■ Give high-flow, high-concentration oxygen by face mask (humidified and warmed to 40–42°C if possible).

TABLE 7.1 ■ *Signs and Symptoms of Hypothermia*

MILD (32–35°C)	MODERATE (28–32°C)	SEVERE (< 28°C)
Slurred speech	Progressively decreased responsiveness	Coma, unresponsive
Mild incoordination	Cyanosis	Dilated and fixed pupils
Shivering	Edema	Ventricular dysrhythmias
Poor judgment	Muscle rigidity, no shivering	Respiratory arrest
	Decreased respiratory rate, bradycardia	

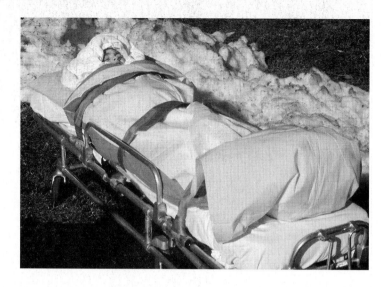

- Assist ventilations with high-flow, high-concentration oxygen when necessary.
- Perform CPR even if no pulse or respirations are present, or follow local protocols or medical direction, based on core body temperature.
- Avoid active external rewarming of the total body so as to prevent a dilation of blood vessels in the extremities. This will cause a secondary drop in core body temperature, hypovolemia, and a fatal heart dysrhythmia. Heat packs may be placed *around the trunk,* but make certain they are not in direct contact with the skin.
- Prevent injuries to cold extremities; wrap extremities with frostbite in warm, dry material; do not rub them or expose them to dry heat.
- Transport patient immediately.
- *DO NOT stop resuscitation in the field. No child is declared dead until warm and dead.*

ALS providers should provide the same care as BLS providers. Do not mechanically stimulate the child with endotracheal intubation, CPR, or suctioning when a heart rate is present (even in severe bradycardia). It is important to prevent the development of ventricular fibrillation, which is difficult to manage in the hypothermic child. Do not waste time in the field to start an IV.

Seizures

A seizure is caused by abnormal bursts of electrical discharge from the brain, leading to periods of involuntary muscle contraction and relaxation, as well as altered mental status. Seizures are caused by a wide variety of disorders, including the following:

- Fever (febrile seizure);
- Epilepsy;
- Inflammation of the brain or its protective lining (encephalitis or meningitis);
- Trauma (birth injury, head trauma, or hypoxic event such as near-drowning);
- Metabolic disorders such as hypoglycemia;

- Poisoning from drugs or lead; and
- Failure to take antiseizure medication.

Seizures are not generally life-threatening unless seizure activity is prolonged, as in the case of *status epilepticus.*

History

Important information to obtain during the history includes the following:

S   How did the child behave when the seizure began (shaking of arms and legs, eyes rolling upward, lip smacking, loss of consciousness, or loss of urinary control)? Has shaking of arms and legs stopped and started up again? Has the child been unconscious the entire time? Does the child respond to voice or touch stimuli even though sleepy? Has there been any difficulty breathing? When did the seizure begin and how long did symptoms last? Does the child have a fever, headache, stiff neck, or other medical illness now?

A   Does the child have any allergies?

M   Does the child take seizure medication? What other medications has the child taken, for example aspirin or acetaminophen (Tylenol)?

P   Has the child previously had a seizure? When was the last seizure? How old was the child when the first seizure occurred? Was this seizure typical of past seizures? Has the child been seen by a physician for any health problem? If so, what was the problem?

L   When was the child's last oral intake? What was it?

E   Were any doses of the child's seizure medications missed recently?

Assessment

The seizure activity will usually be over by the time you arrive at the scene. Children for whom EMS is called will usually be experiencing their first seizure or have a medical illness or an acute head injury that has caused the seizure. In cases of a febrile seizure, the child will have a fever that has risen rapidly, triggering the seizure.

The onset of symptoms is very abrupt, and if this is the child's first seizure, the parents will be alarmed. Signs of a seizure may include any of the following: tonic-clonic movements (sustained muscle contractions in flexion and then extension, followed by alternating muscle contraction and relaxation); loss of consciousness; sudden jerking of a part of the body, such as an arm or a leg (focal seizure); lip smacking; eye blinking; loss of bladder control; staring, or confusion. Following the seizure, the child will be lethargic and sleepy for 5 to 30 minutes.

In cases of status epilepticus, the child has repeated seizures without periods of consciousness so frequently that the child remains unconscious between seizures. This is a true *medical emergency* as the child quickly becomes hypoxic. Sustained seizures without return to consciousness can cause permanent brain damage.

Management

BLS field care for seizures includes the following:

- Monitor the ABCs.
- Position the child on the side if no head or cervical spine injury is suspected. Protect the head and cervical spine if injury to the head or neck could have occurred.

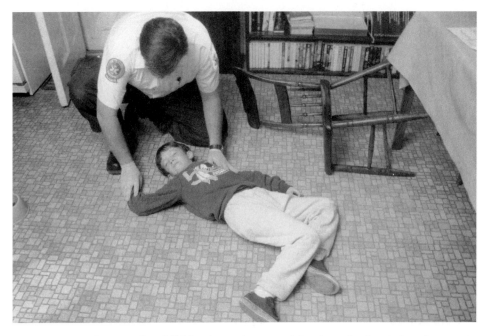

FIGURE 7.2 Protect the child having seizure activity from further injury by moving away furniture or other objects.

- Maintain the child's airway. Do not insert an oral airway or bite block into the mouth; use the jaw-thrust maneuver and suctioning as needed. Children frequently have loose teeth, and one could be knocked out and aspirated.
- Administer high-flow, high-concentration oxygen by mask.
- Protect the child from further injury (Figure 7.2).
- Transport patient immediately.

ALS providers may provide the following additional care under protocol or as ordered by medical direction.

- Endotracheal intubation.
- An IV with Ringer's Lactate or Normal Saline at a keep-open rate.
- 2–4 ml/kg of 25% dextrose in water IV, in case seizure is caused by hypoglycemia.
- Diazepam (Valium) per medical direction orders.

Meningitis

Meningitis can be either a bacterial or viral infection of the central nervous system that is localized in the thin layers (meninges) surrounding the brain and spinal cord. The disorder usually follows an upper airway infection such as an ear infection or tonsillitis.

Approximately 38,000 children develop meningitis each year in the United States. While it occurs in all ages, 90% of cases occur in children between 1 month and 5 years of age. The organism causing meningitis differs by age group. Newborns may develop symptoms within a few days of birth, becoming infected with group B streptococcus bacteria acquired from the mother during delivery. Hemophilus influenzae is the most common bacteria causing meningitis in infants and young children up to 3 years of age. Immunizations for *Hemophilus influenzae* are reducing the number of cases of meningitis in young children from this bacteria.

Meningococcemia (epidemic meningitis) is most common in school-aged children and adolescents.

Bacterial meningitis is life-threatening if antibiotic treatment is delayed. Inflammation of the meninges causes brain swelling and increased intracranial pressure, which leads to altered levels of responsiveness and impaired ventilation. In fact, there is a 5–10% mortality rate in children acquiring bacterial meningitis. Survivors are at high risk for deafness, blindness, retardation, seizure disorders, and learning disabilities.

History

Important information to obtain during the history includes the following:

S Has the baby been extra sleepy and hard to wake up for feeding (For infants < 1 month old)? Has the infant or child been more irritable or hard to console? Has the child's level of responsiveness decreased? Does the child hold the head and neck stiff and resist being held or comforted? Has the child experienced any other symptoms such as vomiting, diarrhea, fever, headache, or respiratory distress? Does the infant or child appear ill? Does the child have a rash that is red, flat, and spreading fast?

A Does the child have any allergies?

M Does the child take any medications? Has the child been given any medication for fever or other symptoms?

P Does the child have any chronic illness? Has the child been treated recently for any health condition, such as an ear infection? What was the health problem?

L What was the child's last oral intake? How long ago was it?

E Has the child been exposed to any serious infection?

Assessment

Signs and symptoms of meningitis are associated with the age of the child (Table 7.2). In all cases the onset of symptoms is abrupt. Some or all of the signs for each age group may be present or develop rapidly as the disease progresses. Any combination of signs should make you more suspicious of meningitis.

The infant or child with meningitis usually has a fever, appears ill, irritable, and does not want to be touched or held. Fever, extra sleepiness, and poor feeding may be the only early signs of meningitis in young infants. Fever and a stiff neck, an altered level of responsiveness, or seizures are often clues to meningitis in older children.

Management

BLS field care for meningitis includes the following:

- Monitor ABCs and vital signs (remember that the infant may develop septic shock or be dehydrated from fever, poor intake, vomiting, and diarrhea).
- Administer high-flow, high-concentration oxygen.
- Provide ventilatory support with a bag-valve mask if needed.
- Prepare for seizures.
- Initiate CPR if indicated.
- Transport patient immediately. (If meningitis is suspected in an infant or a child, be aware that this is considered a true medical emergency. *DO NOT* delay transport.)

TABLE 7.2 ■ *Signs and Symptoms of Meningitis in Infants and Children*

SIGNS AND SYMPTOMS	NEWBORNS/ INFANTS	CHILDREN/ ADOLESCENTS
Fever	± (E)	+, chills (E)
Tachycardia, tachypnea	+	+
Shock	± (L)	± (L)
Unexplained respiratory distress	+ (E)	−
Vomiting	+	+
Diarrhea	±	−
Poor feeding, sucking (may be dehydrated)	+ (E)	−
Seizures	+ (E)	+
Severe headache	−	+ (E)
Irritable, inconsolable	+ (E)	+
Altered mental status	+	+ (E) delirium (L) stupor
Stiff neck	± (L)	± (E)
Arching of back and neck	± (L)	−
High-pitched cry	+	−
Bulging fontanelle	±	−
Petechial rash	−	±

KEY: E, early sign; L, late sign; +, Present; −, Absent; ±, Not always present.

ALS providers should start an IV of Ringer's Lactate or Normal Saline. If the child has hypoperfusion (shock), administer a 20 cc/kg bolus IV push. Repeat the bolus if no improvement in vital signs is noted after 15 minutes. A third bolus may be necessary.

CAUTION!

MENINGOCOCCAL MENINGITIS

If meningococcal meningitis is suspected because a petechial rash is present, you should protect yourself with a gown, gloves, and a mask as soon as possible. Disinfect the unit prior to placing it back in service. If meningococcal meningitis is confirmed, medical evaluation and follow-up is essential for exposed prehospital providers. Antibiotic treatment may be indicated.

Sepsis and Septic Shock

Sepsis is a bacterial infection of the bloodstream, usually occurring as a complication of another infectious site. It is often associated with meningitis. Toxins released by the bacteria may lead to *septic shock.*

Newborns are particularly susceptible to sepsis because their immune systems are not well developed. They become exposed to bacteria either during delivery or in the nursery. Infants and children with chronic illnesses or impaired immune systems are also highly susceptible to sepsis.

History

Important information to obtain during the history includes the following:

S Has the infant or child had any illness, such as vomiting, diarrhea, or fever, in the past week? How has the infant or child been behaving or eating? Is the child more irritable or less responsive than usual? Does the child have pallor, mottling, or cyanosis? Does the infant or child appear ill?

A Does the child have any known allergies?

M Does the child take any medications? Has the child taken any medications for symptoms?

P Does the child have any chronic illness? Has the child been seen recently for any health problem? What was the problem?

L When was the child's last oral intake? What was it?

E Has the child been exposed to any serious infection?

Assessment

Signs and symptoms of sepsis in the newborn and infant are not related to a specific site of infection. They include the following:

- Fever (if present in an infant under 2 months of age, sepsis or meningitis is assumed); however, more commonly, fever is not present.
- Nonspecific respiratory distress (apnea; irregular, grunting respirations; and retractions).
- Vomiting, diarrhea, abdominal distension.
- Poor sucking and feeding.
- Cyanosis, pallor, or mottled skin; there may be jaundice.
- Acute changes in mental status (irritability, tremors, seizures, altered level of responsiveness).
- Signs of increased intracranial pressure if meningitis develops.

Signs of sepsis in an older child include: fever, chills, vomiting or diarrhea, pallor, ill appearance, increased lethargy, and tachycardia.

Septic shock is a life-threatening complication of sepsis, with a high mortality rate in children. Toxins produced by the bacteria cause a dilatation of the peripheral blood vessels and pooling of blood in the extremities. The resulting decreased blood flow to the heart leads to decreased tissue perfusion and plasma leakage from the capillaries. The onset of hypoperfusion (shock) is rapid and can lead to death within a few hours. Signs of hypoperfusion (shock) include the following:

- Altered level of responsiveness—confusion to coma;
- Cool, or cold and clammy skin;
- Tachycardia;
- Prolonged capillary refill time;
- Tachypnea to respiratory failure; and
- Hypotension.

Management

BLS field care for an infant or a child with sepsis and septic shock includes the following:

- Administer high-flow, high-concentration oxygen.
- Monitor ABCs and vital signs.
- Prepare for respiratory and cardiac arrest.

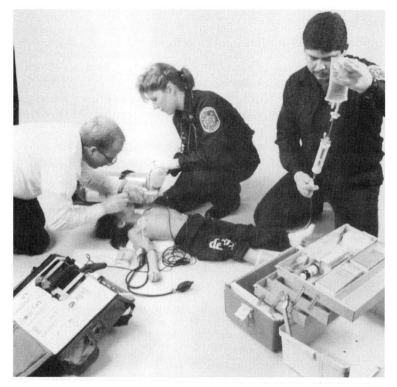

FIGURE 7.3 *Advanced life support for the child in septic shock incudes intubation, assisted ventilation, and IV fluid administration of Ringer's Lactate or Normal Saline in boluses of 20 cc/kg IV push.*

- Transport patient immediately and notify the receiving hospital. *This is a true medical emergency.* As soon as your assessment leads you to suspect sepsis, transport should begin.
- Obtain further history en route.

The ALS provider should provide the following additional care (Figure 7.3):

- Start an IV en route with Ringer's Lactate or Normal Saline and give a bolus of fluid, 20 cc/kg IV push. If vital signs do not stabilize, repeat the fluid bolus.
- Perform endotracheal intubation and provide assisted ventilation when the child becomes less responsive.

Dehydration

Dehydration is an acute loss of body fluids resulting from an imbalance between fluid intake and output. Water (body fluid) is normally lost from 4 systems in the body:

1. The skin by sweating;
2. The respiratory tract to humidify the air breathed;
3. The gastrointestinal tract in the stool and vomitus; and
4. The kidneys in urine.

Dehydration can be a true medical emergency in all age groups, but it tends to strike infants more frequently. Infants are more susceptible to dehydration than adults because a greater proportion of their body is water and their fluid maintenance needs are higher. (See Table 7.3 for a distribution of body fluids by age group.) Severity of dehydration (mild,

TABLE 7.3 ■ *Distribution of Body Fluids by Age Group*

FLUID CHARACTERISTICS	NEWBORN	INFANT (1 YEAR)	ADULT
Weight: lb (kg)	7.5 (3)	22 (10)	154 (70)
Percent of total weight that is water	78	65	60
Percent of body fluids replaced every 24 hours	45	25	20

Source: Adapted from Hochman, H.I., et al. (1979): "Dehydration, diabetic ketoacidosis, and shock in the pediatric patient," *Pediatric Clinics of North America,* 26(4): 804.

moderate, and severe) is based upon the percentage of fluid lost (determined from body weight loss) and signs and symptoms exhibited by the child (Table 7.4).

Infants and children need different amounts of fluid each day to maintain their intake and output balance.

- Infants up to 10 kg need 100 ml/kg of fluid.
- Children between 10 and 20 kg need 1000 ml plus 50 ml for each kg over 10 kg.
- Children over 20 kg need 1500 ml plus 20 ml for each kg over 20 kg.

For example, an infant weighing 9 kg needs 900 ml, an infant weighing 14 kg needs 1200 ml, and a child weighing 26 kg needs 1620 ml of fluid each day.

Acute medical illnesses and sometimes diet interfere with the balance between intake and output in the following ways:

- A fever is associated with increased fluid loss from sweating and tachypnea. At the same time, a child may refuse food and fluids, further jeopardizing the balance.
- Viral gastrointestinal disorders, vomiting, and diarrhea may cause rapid dehydration, especially if oral fluids stimulate further vomiting.
- Diabetic ketoacidosis results in dehydration as the kidneys attempt to flush the high concentration of glucose from the blood.
- Errors in infant formula preparation (making it too concentrated) will result in dehydration as fluid is drawn from cell spaces to dilute the formula in the intestines.

TABLE 7.4 ■ *Classification of Dehydration*

	PERCENT OF BODY WEIGHT LOST	
DEHYDRATION SEVERITY	INFANTS	CHILDREN/ADULTS
Mild	0–5	0–4
Moderate	5–10	4–8
Severe	10–15	8–13

History

Important information to obtain during the history includes the following:

S   Has the infant or child had vomiting or diarrhea? How frequently? Has the child had a fever? If the temperature has been taken, what was it? Has the infant or child been more irritable or less responsive than usual? When was the infant's last wet diaper, or when did the child last urinate? Was the diaper as wet as normal? Was the color of the urine pale or dark?

A   Does the child have any known allergies?

M   Does the child take any medications? Have any medications been given for symptoms of this illness, such as aspirin or acetaminophen (Tylenol) for fever?

P   Does the child have any chronic illness or significant health problem?

L   When was the infant's or child's last bottle or oral intake? What type of fluid was offered? How much was offered and how much was consumed (e.g., 4 oz out of 8 oz)? Is this typical for the child? If breastfeeding, was the feeding typical for the infant?

E   Was the child exposed to a child with a similar illness?

Assessment

Assessment of perfusion status is most important in determining the severity of dehydration. Signs and symptoms of dehydration are variable, but they progress as dehydration worsens (Table 7.5). The child with mild dehydration will develop signs and symptoms during progression to moderate

TABLE 7.5 ■ *Signs and Symptoms of Dehydration*

	DEHYDRATION SEVERITY		
ASSESSMENT	MILD	MODERATE	SEVERE
Vital Signs			
Heart rate	normal	increased	bradycardia or tachycardia, > 130/min
Respiratory rate	normal	increased	tachypnea
Blood pressure	normal	normal	hypotensive, systolic < 80 mm Hg
Capillary refill	< 2 seconds	2–3 seconds	> 3 seconds
Mental Status	alert	irritable	lethargic
Skin			
Color	pale	ashen	mottled
Turgor	normal	poor	tenting
Temperature	warm	cool	cool, clammy
Texture	normal	dry	doughy
Fontanelle	flat	depressed	sunken
Mucous Membranes	dry	very dry/± tears	parched/no tears
Eyes	normal	darkened/sunken	sunken/soft
Thirst	thirsty	increased	intense if alert
Urine Output	normal	decreased/concentrated	minimal/very concentrated

dehydration. The child with severe dehydration will look very ill and is in hypovolemic shock with impending circulatory collapse.

Even though the precise severity of dehydration is difficult to determine, an estimate of severity will be possible with information from the history and assessment of the child. You may be called for a child with moderate to severe dehydration, but mild dehydration may be present when summoned for other medication conditions.

Management

BLS field care for *mild to moderate* dehydration includes the following:

- No special management is needed.
- Offer clear oral liquids if the infant or child can tolerate them without vomiting.
- Monitor ABCs and vital signs.
- Transport patients and contact medical direction.

BLS field care for *severe* dehydration includes:

- Monitor ABCs and vital signs.
- Administer high-flow, high-concentration oxygen.
- Prepare to administer CPR.
- *Transport patient immediately* and contact medical direction.

ALS providers should give the following additional care as directed by medical direction or protocol:

- Start an IV and give a bolus of Ringer's Lactate or Normal Saline at a 20 ml/kg IV push. Monitor vital signs for improvement and repeat the bolus if no change in status is apparent within 5 minutes. A third bolus may be needed.
- Intubate the child if mental status deteriorates.

Diabetic Ketoacidosis

Diabetes mellitus is a chronic disease in which the pancreas does not produce insulin. When insulin is not available, glucose, broken down from foods, is not able to enter muscle or fat cells. Glucose builds up in the bloodstream, causing a high blood sugar or hyperglycemia. The body attempts to compensate for hyperglycemia by diluting the sugar in the blood with water from the cells. The kidneys excrete some of the sugar and excess water, leading to frequent urination (polyuria), dehydration, an electrolyte imbalance, and excessive thirst (polydipsia). Onset of Type I diabetes frequently occurs during childhood or adolescence.

Ketoacidosis occurs when cells cannot use glucose for energy and the body alternatively attempts to break down fats to use as energy. Organic acids called ketones are a by-product of fats. An increase in ketones leads to metabolic acidosis and an acetone or fruity odor to the breath. If this condition is not reversed with insulin therapy and fluid replacement, it becomes life-threatening.

History

Ketoacidosis occurs most often in known diabetics; however, it can also occur in children with disease onset. Questions to ask during the history include the following:

S   Does the child have an acute illness, such as fever, vomiting, or diarrhea? What was the child's last blood glucose test or urine test result? How long ago was the test taken? What was the blood sugar and ketone reading? Has the child had a recent change in thirst or hunger? Has the child been urinating more frequently? Has the child's behavior or level of responsiveness changed recently?

A   Does the child have any known allergies?

M   Does the child take insulin? Has the insulin been taken regularly? When was the last time the insulin dose was changed by the doctor? Does the child take any other medications?

P   Is the child a known diabetic? Has the child had previous problems with blood sugar control? Does the child have any other health problems?

L   When was the child's last oral intake? What was it?

E   Has the child been growing rapidly? Has the child had recent prolonged physical activity? Has the child recently experienced an emotional stress?

The balance between food eaten and insulin dosage is often difficult to maintain in children because they are growing and physically active. Their insulin dose is often changed to adjust to these special requirements. Emotional stress and acute illness also contribute to less well-controlled diabetes.

Assessment

Signs and symptoms of hyperglycemia and ketoacidosis are progressive if the insulin dosage is not adjusted. The development of ketoacidosis takes several days in the case of new disease onset or diet and insulin imbalance. However, ketoacidosis may develop rapidly (in several hours) when triggered by an acute illness, especially if fever, vomiting, and diarrhea are present. Specific signs and symptoms associated with each of the stages of diabetic ketoacidosis are listed below.

Early Stage

- Increased thirst;
- Increased urination;
- Weight loss;
- Hyperglycemia—do a blood glucose check if available.

Acute Stage (Dehydration and Early Ketoacidosis)

- Weakness, abdominal pain, generalized aches;
- Loss of appetite; nausea and vomiting;
- Signs of dehydration, except frequent urination, may continue because of the kidney's response to hyperglycemia;
- Fruity or acetone breath odor;
- Tachypnea, hyperventilation to blow off CO_2, tachycardia.

Precomatose Stage: Ketoacidosis

- Altered mental status (responsive to verbal or pain stimuli);
- Tachypnea, tachycardia;
- Nausea, vomiting, abdominal pain;
- Signs of moderate dehydration.

Comatose Stage

- Deep and slow respirations (Kussmaul);
- Signs of severe dehydration;
- Tachycardia, weak pulse;
- Hypotension;
- Rigid abdomen.

Management

BLS field care for diabetic ketoacidosis includes the following:

- Monitor ABCs and vital signs.
- Protect the airway, preventing aspiration if vomiting occurs.
- Should the child have hypoglycemia rather than early diabetic ketoacidosis, give oral fluids with sugar if the patient is *alert* and able to swallow (Figure 7.4).
- Administer high-flow, high-concentration oxygen by face mask and assist ventilations as needed.
- Transport patient promptly.

ALS providers may additionally start an IV with Ringer's Lactate or Normal Saline, administering a 20 ml/kg bolus IV push, and repeating the bolus if no change in vital signs is apparent. Intubate the child if the mental status deteriorates.

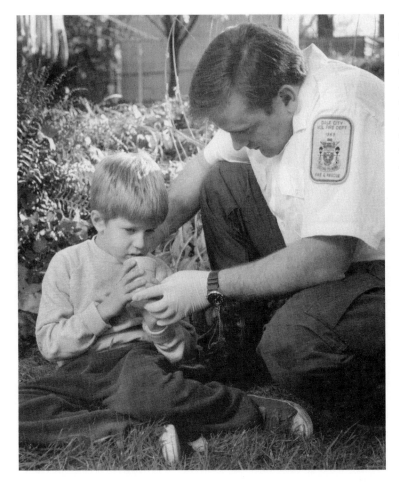

FIGURE 7.4 *When a diabetic child develops symptoms of early diabetic ketoacidosis or hypoglycemia and no blood sugar test is available, give oral fluids with sugar. Until the child gets to the hospital, it is more important to manage hypoglycemia, which may become life-threatening, than to worry about increasing the child's blood sugar.*

Hypoglycemia

Hypoglycemia, or low blood glucose level, in the prehospital setting is usually a problem associated with known diabetics and newborn infants. It can be as life-threatening as hyperglycemia, and if not promptly treated, can result in permanent brain damage. Causes of hypoglycemia in known diabetics can result from either an:

- Increase in exercise without adequate food intake or a reduction in prescribed insulin, or
- Increase in administered insulin, whether accidental or intentional without additional food intake.

History

Important questions to ask during the history include the following:

S Did the child feel weak or dizzy very suddenly? Has there been a sudden change in behavior, such as anxiety, mood swings, or irritability? Is the child breathing rapidly or having difficulty breathing? Has a blood sugar test been taken in the last few minutes? What was the reading?

A Does the child have any known allergies?

M Was there a change in the amount or type of insulin administered just prior to symptoms? Has the child been taking any other medications?

P Is the child a known diabetic? Does the child have any other health problems?

L When was the child's last oral intake? Was any juice or sugar given when the symptoms occurred?

E Has the child recently changed daily exercise routine or sports involvement?

Assessment

Children with *mild hypoglycemia* generally have feelings of hunger, weakness, as well as a rapid respiratory rate and heart rate.

Children with *moderate hypoglycemia* will have more severe symptoms such as sweating, tremors, anxiety, irritability, vomiting, and mood swings. They may complain of a stomachache, headache, dizziness, or blurring of vision.

Children with *severe hypoglycemia* have a decreased level of responsiveness to verbal or painful stimuli only, seizures, tachycardia, and hypoperfusion (shock).

It is very difficult to determine the difference between hypoglycemia and hyperglycemia symptoms in children. Prehospital providers who carry blood glucose test strips should check the blood glucose level prior to initiating management. Because hypoglycemia may be life-threatening if not treated promptly, treatment is initiated (even when blood glucose test strips are not available) when it is strongly suspected.

Management

BLS field care for hypoglycemia includes the following:

- Monitor ABCs and vital signs.
- Assessment may include a blood glucose test when available.
- Give oral fluid with sugar or oral glucose by mouth when child is alert and able to swallow.

■ *Transport patient immediately* when there is an altered mental status or when there is no response to sugar or oral glucose.

ALS providers should perform the following additional care as directed by medical direction or protocols:

■ Start an IV with Ringer's Lactate or Normal Saline and then administer a bolus of 25% dextrose 2–4 cc/kg (0.5–1.0 g/kg) IV push. (The 50% dextrose should be diluted with sterile water in a 1:1 concentration. The 25% concentration is less irritating to the child's veins.)

■ If IV access is not possible, administer glucagon IM (when available), 0.03–0.1 mg/kg per dose. It may be repeated in 20 minutes as necessary.

■ When available, repeat the blood glucose test 10–15 minutes following dextrose infusion to determine a response.

Anaphylaxis

Anaphylaxis is a rare, acute, and generalized allergic reaction. The reaction may occur within minutes to hours after an exposure to the substance by ingestion, inhalation, or injection. Common substances triggering this allergic response include bee stings, antibiotics, drugs, and foods (Figure 7.5). Generally, the child has had one prior exposure to the substance, at which time the child became "sensitive." Subsequent exposures to the same substance result in the severe allergic reaction.

Generally, four body systems are affected—skin, respiratory system, cardiovascular system, and gastrointestinal tract. However, the response is individual to the patient. Any or all systems can be affected initially.

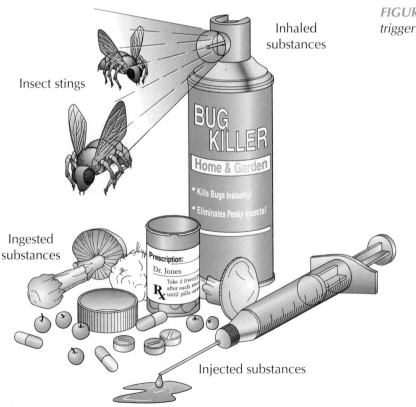

FIGURE 7.5   Common substances that trigger anaphylactic allergic responses.

History

Important questions to ask during assessment and transport of the patient include the following:

S Is the child having any difficulty breathing? Does the child have a rash, hives, or other swelling? How much time was there between exposure and onset of symptoms? (The more rapid the reaction, the more severe the shock.) Is the child anxious? Has the child's level of responsiveness decreased?

A Does the child have any known allergies? What was the possible substance (food, bee sting, drug, etc.) that triggered this reaction?

M Does the child have an epi-pen (preloaded epinephrine) for such allergic reactions? Has it already been injected? If so, how long ago? If not, is it available?

P Is there a prior history of anaphylaxis or serious allergic reactions? Does the child have any other health problems?

L When was the child's last oral intake? What was it?

E Was the child in an environment that could have resulted in exposure?

Assessment

During the initial assessment, look for signs of respiratory distress and altered mental status. When you arrive at the scene, the child may be in acute distress with shock and an airway obstruction. Look for a medic alert tag. Signs of a generalized reaction by body system include:

- *Skin*—hives, itching, and redness; swelling of the face, mouth, and tongue.
- *Respiratory*—wheezing, respiratory distress, and tightness in the chest; stridor, choking, and hoarseness.
- *Gastrointestinal*—nausea and vomiting; diarrhea and abdominal cramps.
- *Circulatory*—flushed skin; tachycardia, bradycardia, and/or cardiac arrest.
- *Neurologic*—seizures, loss of bladder and bowel control.

Management

BLS management for anaphylaxis includes the following steps:

- Monitor ABCs and vital signs.
- Administer high-flow, high-concentration oxygen.
- Prepare to administer rescue breathing and CPR.
- If patient carries epinephrine for anaphylaxis and has not yet injected it, inject it or assist the patient or family member in administering it.
- Transport the child rapidly to the emergency department.
- If the allergy results from a bee sting or other injected venom, delay the absorption of the substance with a cold pack over the site.
- If hypotension is present, the child should be placed with legs raised to a 30-degree angle.

ALS providers should provide the following additional care:

- Perform endotracheal intubation. Remember that the endotracheal tube may need to be a size or two smaller than usual because of laryngeal edema.
- Initiate cardiac monitoring and pulse oximetry if available.

- Start an IV of Ringer's Lactate or Normal Saline. Administer a bolus of fluid IV push, 20 ml/kg. If there is no change in vital signs after the first bolus of fluid and epinephrine administration, the bolus of fluid can be repeated.
- For severe reactions, medical direction may recommend that epinephrine 1:10,000 be administered IV at a dose of 0.01 mg/kg, very slowly. Monitor for hypertension and bradycardia. If the IV cannot be established, epinephrine can be administered by IO or endotracheal tube. Local protocols or medical direction may recommend repeated doses of epinephrine.
- Alternately, epinephrine 1:1000 (0.01 ml/kg every 15 min $\times$ 3) may be given subcutaneously.
- Administer other drugs per medical direction, such as IV diphenhydramine, aminophylline, and dopamine; or nebulized albuterol (0.25 ml of 5% solution in 2.5 ml of Normal Saline).

Congenital Heart Defects

The heart has two circulatory pathways—transporting blood requiring oxygen to the lungs (pulmonary circulation) and transporting oxygenated blood to the major organs and extremities (systemic circulation). In the normal heart without defects, these two circulatory pathways do not allow the two bloods to mix.

Congenital defects of the heart or the aorta and pulmonary artery are the primary cause of heart disease in children. These defects are present, but not always detected, at birth. They are usually detected during infancy and early childhood. The cause of most congenital defects is unknown, although heredity and maternal infection or drug use during pregnancy are associated with such defects.

Heart structures that may be defective include:

- A valve that is too small, does not completely close, or is absent.
- The wall between two heart chambers has an opening where none should exist.
- The aorta and pulmonary artery are improperly formed or in the wrong position.
- The channel between the pulmonary artery and aorta (ductus arteriosis, an important feature of fetal circulation) does not close after birth.

Single or multiple defects can occur. Some defects allow blood in the two circulatory pathways to mix, often resulting in cyanosis. Sometimes the heart is unable to pump effectively because of a congenital defect or other acquired disease. This results in *congestive heart failure,* either because the heart is unable to get enough blood to the body to meet its needs, or it is unable to handle the venous blood return adequately. Infants and children often have different signs of congestive heart failure than adults.

Infants with heart defects that allow the blood to mix and cause cyanosis can develop *hypoxic spells,* or cyanotic spells. These spells occur when the oxygen demand acutely exceeds the oxygen in the blood, leading to metabolic acidosis. Usually, the spells occur in the morning, after feeding or crying. They progress to seizures, stroke, or even death if not rapidly treated.

History

When the EMS is called for these children, the parents know the child has a heart defect. In these instances, specific information to obtain during the history includes the following:

S Has the child's feeding pattern changed? Is the child more cyanotic than usual? What kind of spell did the child have? What triggered it and how long did it last? Does the child use oxygen and was it used today? What other treatment was given and what was the response?

A Does the child have any known allergies?

M Does the child take any medications such as digoxin or diuretics? Did the child take the medication today? Was any other medication given?

P What is the name of the child's heart defect? (to share with medical direction) Has the child had any heart surgery or is surgery planned? When? Was the defect totally corrected?

L When was the child's last oral intake? Does the child use any special feeding device?

E Has the child had any recent illness or stress? What are the child's baseline vital signs if known?

Assessment

A request for assistance and transport will most often occur when the child develops respiratory distress associated with an acute illness, congestive heart failure, or a hypoxic spell.

Signs and symptoms of a hypoxic spell

- Prolonged crying and irritability;
- Rapid and deep respirations;
- Increasing cyanosis, poor tissue perfusion;
- Limpness;
- Loss of consciousness, seizures, cardiac arrest.

Signs and symptoms of congestive heart failure are associated with the side of the heart that is not pumping effectively.

- *Respiratory*—retractions, tachypnea, dyspnea that increases with feedings, crackles or wheezing on auscultations, cough.
- *Circulatory*—tachycardia, delayed capillary refill, weak peripheral pulses, heart murmur.
- *Neurologic*—decreased responsiveness, irritability when disturbed, limpness of extremities.
- *Skin*—pallor or cyanosis; cool, moist skin; noticeable sweating, puffy eyes.
- *General*—fatigue and exhaustion, small and poorly developed for age.

Management

BLS field care for the infant or child with a cardiac emergency includes:

- Monitor ABCs and vital signs.
- Maintain the airway.
- Administer high-flow, high-concentration oxygen.
- Assist ventilations as necessary.
- Calm the child.

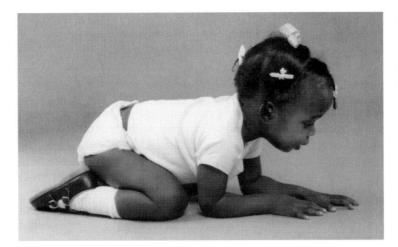

FIGURE 7.6 *Place the infant having a "cyanotic spell" in knee-chest position. This will decrease the blood flow from the legs to the heart and reduce the heart's workload temporarily.*

- For a hypoxic spell, place the child in knee-chest position (Figure 7.6).
- Prepare to assist ventilations.
- Prepare for cardiopulmonary arrest.
- *Transport patient immediately.*

The ALS provider should initiate the following additional care:

- Start an IV with D5W at a keep-open rate if there is an anticipated lengthy transport time if directed by local protocol or medical direction.
- Attach a cardiac monitor and pulse oximeter if available.
- Administer medications according to medical direction.

Children Assisted by High-Technology Equipment

Children with a wide variety of chronic illnesses are often cared for at home by parents. Some of the conditions that these children have include the following: respiratory and cardiac disabling conditions, feeding disorders, disabilities associated with severe trauma, and terminal illnesses.

These children are at home primarily because of benefits to the child, family, and the health care system. The home is a more positive environment for the child to grow and develop than is a hospital intensive care unit. However, families take on a tremendous burden to care for the child at home, often disrupting the lives of all family members. Parents are often exhausted caring for the child 24 hours a day. They often have no relief because other family members and baby-sitters are afraid to care for the child.

The *respiratory disabled* include such children as premature babies who require life-saving, long-term mechanical ventilation. Surviving babies often develop a chronic lung disease characterized by hypoxia, hypercarbia, and oxygen dependence. Advanced cystic fibrosis is another respiratory disorder sometimes requiring technology assistance. Such children will have signs of respiratory distress with crackles, wheezes, abundant secretions, retractions, and cyanosis on exertion. These children may be treated at home with any of the following adjuncts: oxygen, mechanical ventilators, suction, tracheostomies, and apnea monitors.

Cardiac disabled infants and children include those with congenital cardiac defects who are waiting for surgery or have a defect that cannot be surgically corrected. They will have signs of hypoxia, decreased exercise tolerance, and sometimes congestive heart failure. These children are treated at home with oxygen and feeding pumps.

Children with major *trauma disabilities* that are the result of a head or spinal cord injury or near-drowning are often treated at home after discharge from a rehabilitation hospital. They may be on life-support equipment such as oxygen, mechanical ventilators, suction, and feeding pumps. Some of these children will have a gastrostomy tube that permits tube-feeding directly into the stomach or a central line type of Broviac catheter for IV nutrition.

Some children receive hospice care at home for a terminal illness. Rather than life-support equipment, these children will have equipment necessary for comfort measures, such as IV pumps for drug administration. Families of children with terminal illness made the decision to permit the child to die at home rather than in the hospital. EMS will not usually be called to administer care to these children unless the family has not resolved the issue of the child's death. When EMS is called, providers are required to begin resuscitation unless special "do not resuscitate" provisions are part of local protocols. Often the local EMS agency is notified about the child in the community so an appropriate priority can be place on emergency care.

Reasons Why EMS Is Activated

Prehospital care providers are generally called to help these families in times of crisis. EMS providers are often notified about the child in the community by the family or health care providers. While parents have been well trained to manage all types of problems, the child might become acutely ill, equipment might fail, or the parent might panic because of fatigue. Examples of some of these problems include the following:

- Severe respiratory distress or respiratory arrest;
- The tracheostomy tube has become obstructed and the parent is unable to clear it or change it; or
- The child has hemorrhaged.

Management

BLS and ALS field care should include the following:

- Assess and manage the ABCs.
- Treat parents as you would another health professional. They are experienced in treating their child's condition and know the critical information you need about changes in the child's status.
- Parents may already be providing emergency care (CPR, assisted ventilation, suctioning, etc.), so support their efforts. It is not always necessary to take over for the parents.
- When an equipment malfunction has occurred, attach the child to your equipment, rather than try to determine what is wrong with the child's equipment. Vendors will repair the equipment.
- Provide rapid transport to the hospital, notifying the hospital to contact the child's physician.
- When transporting children who use assistive devices (wheelchairs, communication boards, hearing aids, glasses, etc.) take these items with the child. They often facilitate emergency care.

Medical Emergencies References

Ball, J., and Bindler, R., *Pediatric Nursing: Caring for Children.* Norwalk, CT: Appleton & Lange, 1995.

Baraff, L.J., Bass, J.W., Fleisher, G.R., et al., "Practice guidelines for the management of infants and children 0 to 36 months of age with fever without source," *Annals of Emergency Medicine,* 22, no. 7 (July 1993), pp. 1198–1210.

Brown, K., "Septic shock: How to stop the deadly cascade," *American Journal of Nursing,* 94, no. 9 (September 1994), pp. 20–27.

———. "Critical interventions in septic shock," *American Journal of Nursing,* 94, no. 10 (October 1994), pp. 20–26.

Cason, D., "Anaphylactic shock," *JEMS,* 14, no. 2 (February 1989), pp. 42–46, 51.

Chameides, L., and Hazinski, M.F., eds., *Textbook of Pediatric Advanced Life Support,* 2nd ed. Dallas: American Heart Association, 1994.

Clark, J., and Starr-McNamara, L., "Heart disease: More than just blue babies," *JEMS,* 10, (1993), pp. 37–43.

Coffman, S.P., "Home care of the child and family after near-drowning," *Journal of Pediatric Health Care,* 6, no. 1 (January/February 1992), pp. 18–24.

Corey, E.C., "Treatment for anaphylaxis," *Emergency,* 25, no. 10 (October 1993) pp. 48–59.

Cox, D., "Diazepam use for seizures," *Emergency,* 25, no. 9 (September 1993), pp. 20–27, 66–67.

———. "Seizures and epilepsy: Understanding the differences," *Emergency,* 26, no. 9 (September 1994), pp. 32–35.

Crabb, T.J., "In the hot seat: Managing febrile seizures," *JEMS,* 18, no. 1 (January 1993), pp. 50–56.

DeBoer, S., "The case of the blue baby: ED management of tetralogy of Fallot," *Journal of Emergency Nursing,* 22, no. 1 (February 1996), pp. 73–76.

Duggan, C., Santosham, M., and Glass, R., "The management of acute diarrhea in children: Oral rehydration, rehydration maintenance, and nutritional therapy," *MMWR,* 41, RR-16, (1992), pp. 1–20.

Feigin, R.D., McCracken, G.H., and Klein, J.O., "Diagnosis and management of meningitis," *Pediatric Infectious Disease,* 11, no. 9 (September 1992), pp. 785–814.

Gildea, J.H., "When fever is the enemy," *Pediatric Nursing,* 18, no. 2 (March/April 1992), pp. 165–167.

Henderson, D.P., and Brownstein, D., eds., *Pediatric Emergency Nursing Manual.* New York: Springer Publishing Co., 1994.

Hochman, H.I., et al., "Dehydration, diabetic ketoacidosis, and shock in the pediatric patient," *Pediatric Clinics of North America,* 26, no. 4 (November 1979), pp. 803–825.

Israel, R.S., "Endocrine and metabolic emergencies: Diabetic ketoacidosis," *Emergency Medical Clinics of North America,* 7, no. 4 (November 1989) pp. 859–871.

Park, M.K., Pediatric *Cardiology for Practitioners,* 3rd ed. St. Louis: Mosby Year Book, Inc., 1996.

Saez-Llorens, X., and McCracken, G.H., "Sepsis syndrome and septic shock in pediatrics: Current concepts of terminology, pathophysiology, and management," *Journal of Pediatrics,* 123, no. 4 (October 1993), pp. 497–508.

Singer, J.I., Vest, J., and Prints, A., "Occult bacteremia and septicemia in the febrile child younger than 2 years," *Emergency Clinics of North America,* 13, no. 2 (May 1995), pp. 381–416.

Stenklyft, P.H., and Carmona, M., "Febrile seizures," *Emergency Clinics of North America,* 12, no. 4 (November 1995) pp. 989–999.

Throckmorton, D.W., Throckmorton, K., and Montgomery, J.R., "Self-defense: Precautions for pediatric infectious diseases," *Emergency,* 23, no. 8 (August 1991), pp. 42–45, 54.

Vining, E.P.G., "Pediatric seizures," *Emergency Clinics of North America,* 12, no. 4 (November 1994), pp. 973–988.

Wertz, W., "On guard for meningitis," *Emergency,* 27, no. 8 (August 1995), pp. 36–39.

Poisoning Emergencies

OBJECTIVES

When you have completed this chapter you should be able to

▶ Describe the contribution of developmental stage to childhood poisoning.
▶ List signs of toxins on various body systems.
▶ List important information to collect at the scene of a poisoning emergency.
▶ Describe poisoning emergencies in which vomiting should be induced.
▶ Demonstrate field management of the child with a poisoning emergency.

Developmental Considerations

In 1994, nearly 1.9 million cases of poisonings were reported to U.S. poison control centers nationwide. Children accounted for 67.8% of all cases reported. More boys than girls were victims in children under 13 years of age, but this frequency reversed itself in adolescents. More than 90% of all poisoning events occurred in the home (Table 8.1). Only 9.8% of toxic exposures in children under 20 years of age resulted in death, and of these, 58.7% of all child fatalities occurred in the 13-to-19-year age group. (Litovitz et al., 1994)

Poisoning is a major cause of preventable death in children under 5 years of age, with a peak incidence in children between 2 and 3 years of age. This age group is at greater risk for poisoning because of certain developmental characteristics (Figure 8.1).

- They explore by putting objects in their mouth.
- Taste is not well developed, so they will drink or eat (ingest) seemingly distasteful liquids and other substances.
- They are becoming more independent, mobile, and curious.
- Their fine motor skills have developed so they can open drawers, closets, and most containers.
- They cannot read labels, and many drugs look like candy.

The Poison Prevention Packaging Act of 1970 has helped reduce the incidence of poisoning by requiring child safety caps on all potentially toxic substances and drugs. The caps are designed to *delay* access to the substance by a child under 4 years of age. However, children still get access to toxic substances for the following reasons:

- Child safety caps are not replaced properly on containers.
- A nonsafety cap is requested for a drug at the pharmacy.
- Substances are put in different containers without safety caps, such as paint thinner in a soda bottle.
- Substances are packaged in containers similar to those used for food, such as milk and bleach both in plastic bottles.

TABLE 8.1 ■ *The Number and Percentage of Poisonings by Age Group Reported to Poison Control Centers in 1994*

AGE GROUPS	NUMBER OF POISONINGS (%)
< 3 years	774,672 (40.1%)
3–5 years	267,752 (13.8%)
6–12 years	125,397 (6.5%)
13–19 years	137,450 (7.1%)
20–99 years	604,738 (31.4%)
Total children < 20 years	1,305,271 (67.8%)
Total all ages	1,926,438 (31.4%)

Source: Adapted from Litovitz, T.L., et al., (1995): "1994 Annual Report of the American Association of Poison Control Centers Toxic Exposure Surveillance System," *American Journal of Emergency Medicine,* 13(5): 551–597.

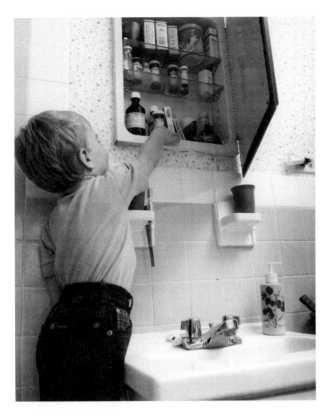

FIGURE 8.1 Children between 2 and 3 years of ages are at great risk of poisoning because of their exploring behavior.

Toxic substances that young children often ingest include the following:

- Over-the-counter medications such as cough and cold preparations, vitamins, topical skin care preparations, and gastrointestinal preparations;
- Cosmetics and personal care products;
- Household cleaners;
- Analgesics such as aspirin, acetaminophen, ibuprofen, and narcotics;
- Plants such as pepper, philodendron, poinsettias, holly, and dumbcane.

Toxic substances that school-age children and adolescents ingest, in order of frequency, as reported to poison control centers in 1994 included the following:

- Analgesics;
- Over-the-counter medications of the same types ingested by young children;
- Insecticides and pesticides;
- Household cleaners;
- Cosmetics and personal care products.

School-age children and adolescents often experiment with various drugs, and they may unintentionally take an overdose. They are curious about the effect of various drugs and are greatly influenced by their peers to use drugs recreationally. These children use drugs to get "high," to experience perceptual and sensory sensations. Some children experiment with drugs as part of a social group (peer pressure), sharing the experience and feeling as though they are getting away with something by breaking the rules (Figure 8.2). This misuse may lead to substance abuse and even addiction to some drugs.

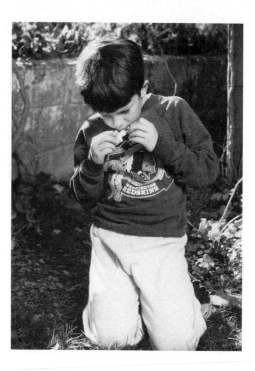

FIGURE 8.2 Older children often experiment to experience the feelings associated with inhaling substances.

Marijuana is the most widely used illicit drug among adolescents. At some point in the past year, 11.7% of 8th graders, 25% of 10th graders, and 31% of 12th graders have used it at least once. Inhalants are the second most common illicit drug used by adolescents. The use of alcohol and cigarettes is even more common among adolescents, with 80% of all students using alcohol at least once by the 12th grade. More than half (56%) of 8th graders report trying alcohol, and 25% are current drinkers. (Johnston, et al., 1995)

Chronic drug use and drug dependence may be the result of children who have other motivations. Such motivations may include seeking the following:

- An escape from reality or from problems;
- An escape from feelings of anger, depression, and disenchantment with the adult world;
- Feelings of power, excitement, and confidence.

In 1994, nearly 50% of poisonings in adolescents between 13 and 19 years of age were intentional. Drug overdose may be intentional in school-age children and adolescents who are attempting suicide. (See Chapter 16, "Suicide in Children and Adolescents.")

Effect of Toxins on Body Systems

The initial concern in poisonings is whether the drug will quickly depress the respiratory system, leading to respiratory arrest. Depending upon the type of substance, various systems will be affected directly or through complications caused by the toxic substance. Some poisons cause life-threatening symptoms in the respiratory, circulatory, and central nervous systems. The gastrointestinal system is often burned and irritated by the corrosive substance ingested, such as drain cleaners, dishwasher detergent, toilet bowl cleaners, and other concentrated cleansers (Table 8.2).

TABLE 8.2 ■ *Effect of Various Poisonous Substances on Body Systems**

DRUG/POISON	RESPIRATORY SYSTEM	CIRCULATORY SYSTEM	NERVOUS SYSTEM	GASTROINTESTINAL SYSTEM
Alcohol (A) *Barbiturates* (B) *Sedatives*	Depressed rate	Tachycardia, first Bradycardia Low blood pressure	Aggression Violence ↓ coordination ↓ perception Slurred speech Loss of inhibitions (A) Constricted pupils (B)	
Amphetamines Cocaine Hallucinogens	↑ rate	Tachycardia ↑ blood pressure Dysrhythmias	Euphoria Agitation Restlessness Dilated pupils Seizures	
Digitalis (D) *Beta-blockers*		Bradycardia (D) Dysrhythmias		
Narcotics	Depressed rate	Bradycardia ↓ blood pressure	Euphoria, first Lethargy Loss of consciousness Constricted pupils	
Anticholinergics (atropine)	↑ rate	Tachycardia ↑ blood pressure		
Aspirin	↑ rate (metabolic acidosis)	Hypoperfusion (shock) GI bleeding	Fever	Abdominal pain Nausea, vomiting
Hydrocarbons (e.g. kerosene)	↑ rate, distress (with aspiration)			Abdominal pain Nausea, vomiting
Organophosphates (e.g. fertilizer)	↑ rate, wheezing		Seizures, fever Pinpoint pupils	Vomiting, drooling, ↑ salivation
Corrosive substances (e.g. lye)	Obstruction	Hypoperfusion (shock)		Drooling ↑ salivation Abdominal pain Nausea, vomiting Burns to mouth
Organic solvents (inhaled) (e.g. gasoline, airplane glue)			↓ coordination ↓ perception Euphoria Lethargy Loss of consciousness	

*KEY: The capital letter following a sign in a body system indicates the specific sign associated with a drug/poison coded with the same capital letter.

Effect of Toxins on Body Systems

History

Important information to obtain during the hisrory includes the following:

S   What symptoms does the child have? Has the child's behavior changed, for example, more restless or agitated? Has the child vomited? If so, was it induced or did it occur spontaneously? Is the child complaining of nausea or abdominal pain? Is the child less responsive than usual? Are there any signs of burns or other materials seen around the mouth or on other parts of the body? Is there drooling or increased salivation? Are the pupils dilated or pinpoint?

A   Does the child have any known allergies?

M   Does the child take any medications regularly? Were any special medications given today?

P   Does the child have any significant health problems? If so, what is the problem?

L   When did the child last have an oral intake? What was it?

E   What was taken, how much, and how long ago? Was the substance swallowed, inhaled, injected, or absorbed through the skin? What treatment has been initiated?

Assessment

Upon arriving at the scene, conduct the initial assessment to identify any life-threatening problems. Corrosive substances may cause swelling in the mouth and throat. Look for signs of burns around the mouth. Spontaneous vomiting can occur with any substances swallowed.

The actual signs and symptoms present in the child will vary depending upon both the poisoning substance, mechanism of poisoning (swallowed, inhaled, injected, or absorbed), and the time since the child was exposed. (Refer to Table 8.2 for common signs and symptoms for various groups of poisons.) The child's level of responsiveness may change rapidly, so reassess the child frequently.

Inspect the scene for signs of a mechanism of injury (bottles or containers, plastic bags, traces of substances, injection paraphernalia, plants). Be sure to take any evidence to the hospital for analysis. Any drug paraphernalia should be labeled using chain of possession procedures to give to the police as evidence. Note the general condition of the environment and any signs of poison prevention for the young child.

Management

General BLS care for poisonings include the following:

- Upon arrival at the scene, conduct the initial assessment, identifying any immediately life-threatening problems. Remove the child from an environment of inhalants, while protecting yourself.
- Ensure the airway and protect the cervical spine if head or neck injury could have occurred. Be prepared for aggressive airway management.
- Continually reassess the child's ABCDEs and vital signs.
- Using gloves, remove any pills or other substances from the child's mouth.
- Call the poison control center or medical direction for specific treatment. State the signs and symptoms noted in the child and give any specific information about the toxin that is known. *In some states,*

the poison control center has no medical director, and local medical direction must be consulted prior to initiating management.

- For substances with a hydrocarbon, caustic, or corrosive base, follow guidelines for administration of activated charcoal from the poison control center or local medical direction. (See also Caution box, page 142.) In cases of corrosives, initially dilute the toxin with milk or water to prevent further damage.
- Administer high-flow, high-concentration oxygen by mask and closely monitor for vomiting. Oxygen can help reverse decreased responsiveness, especially in cases of respiratory depression or carbon monoxide poisoning.
- Assist ventilations in cases of decreasing levels of responsiveness. Prepare to perform CPR if the child's mental status continues to deteriorate.
- Transport rapidly and contact medical direction. Bring all containers, toxic substances, and vomitus to the hospital.

ALS providers should consider the following additional management procedures for the child who has decreased responsiveness, seizures, or coma resulting from a poison:

- Perform endotracheal intubation in cases of decreased responsiveness, especially as the gag reflex disappears.
- Start an IV with Ringer's Lactate or Normal Saline at a keep-open rate, unless signs of hypoperfusion (shock) are present. If shock is present, administer a 20 ml/kg bolus IV push and repeat if no change in vital signs is apparent.
- Administer dextrose 0.5–1.0 g/kg/IV dose (2–4 ml/kg/D25W) if no mechanism of injury is present. Check the blood glucose level first whenever possible.
- Administer naloxone 0.1 mg/kg per dose IV initially to a maximum dose of 2 mg. If there is no response in 10 minutes, then give 2 mg IV if a narcotic overdose is suspected.
- Administer atropine 0.02–0.05 mg/kg per dose IV if an organophosphate poisoning is suspected. The dose can be repeated every 10 to 15 minutes to a maximum of 2 mg.

Guidelines for Use of Activated Charcoal

Activated charcoal is an agent that binds poisons to the gastrointestinal tract to prevent their absorption into the bloodstream. It can be used alone for most ingested poisons, but it is not effective for iron, alcohols, and strong acid and alkali substances.

Prior to giving activated charcoal, assess the child's level of responsiveness and consider if decreased responsiveness may occur over the next 20 minutes. Give 1 g/kg premixed to the child to drink. If powdered charcoal is used, taste can be improved by mixing it with fruit juice or chocolate powder and water. Do not mix it with milk products as this decreases its binding capacity. Place the charcoal solution in a covered cup and use a straw so the child is less likely to resist drinking it (Figure 8.3). For children with decreased responsiveness, ALS providers may administer the activated charcoal by nasogastric tube.

Guidelines for Use of Syrup of Ipecac

While there is still some controversy, syrup of ipecac is sometimes used to induce vomiting in cases of swallowed poisons to reduce the amount of

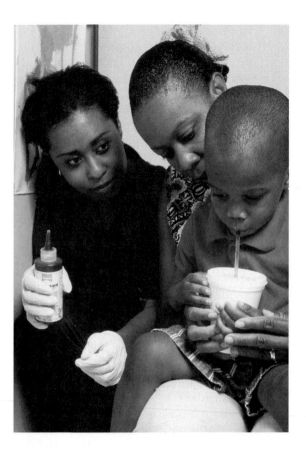

FIGURE 8.3 *Administration of activated charcoal after ingestion of a poison.*

poison absorbed into the bloodstream through the gastrointestinal tract. Many parents are still encouraged to keep syrup of ipecac on hand in case of a poisoning. It is less common for prehospital providers to administer it. Medical direction may recommend inducing vomiting for the child who has ingested a hydrocarbon compound (organophosphate pesticide, camphor, or heavy metals) containing a substance more harmful to the central nervous system than the effects caused by aspirating the hydrocarbon.

Syrup of ipecac takes approximately 20 minutes to induce vomiting. The dosage is dependent upon age: 10 ml to infants between 6 and 12 months of age; 15 ml to children between 1 and 12 years of age; and 30 ml to children over 12 years of age. Once ipecac is given, have the child drink 8 oz of water, which dilutes the poison and stimulates vomiting. If the child does not vomit in 20 minutes, the dose can be repeated if the child's level of responsiveness is not expected to decrease.

CAUTION!

Contraindications to the use of ipecac include the following:

- decreased responsiveness;
- no gag reflex;
- under 6 months of age;
- ingestion of a petroleum distillate, strong acid or alkali product, or a rapid acting central nervous system agent;
- cervical spine injury; and
- increased vagal tone.

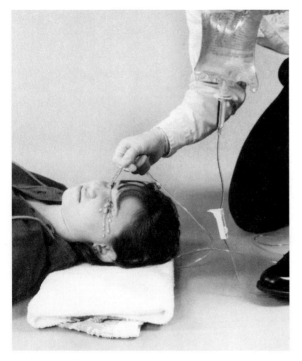

FIGURE 8.4 *Flushing the eye to remove any poisons.*

Poisons on the Skin or in the Eyes

BLS care for the child with poisons *absorbed by the skin* includes the following:

- Clothing should be removed as the child is flushed with copious amounts of water. The prehospital provider should wear gloves and eye protection to avoid exposure.
- Any poisons in direct contact with the eyes should be flushed for 15 to 20 minutes, using water or saline. Hold the child's head over the sink or tub and pour the solution directly into the eye. Avoid draining into the unaffected eye (Figure 8.4). During transport, use IV solution with the end of the IV tubing used to direct the solution away from the unaffected eye.
- Refer to the management of chemical burns in Chapter 12, "Burns."

Poisoning Emergencies References

Ball, J.W., and Bindler, R., *Pediatric Nursing: Caring for Children.* Norwalk, CT: Appleton & Lange, 1995, pp. 533–536.

Bond, G.R., "The poisoned child: Evolving concepts in care," *Emergency Clinics of North America,* 13, no. 2 (May 1995), pp. 343–355.

Committee on Injury and Poison Prevention, *Handbook of Common Poisonings in Children.* Elk Grove, IL: American Academy of Pediatrics, 1994, pp. 27–29.

Corey, E.C., "The treatment of poisonings," *Emergency,* 26, no 2 (February 1994), pp. 20–26.

Johnston, L.D., O'Malley, P.M., and Bachman, J.G., *National Survey Results on Drug Use from the Monitoring of the Future Study, 1975–1994, Vol 1: Secondary School Students.* Rockville, MD: National Institute on Drug Abuse, NIH Pub. No. 95-4026, 1995.

Litovitz, T.L., et al., "1994 Annual Report of the American Association of Poison

Control Centers Toxic Exposure Surveillance System," *American Journal of Emergency Medicine*, 13, no. 5 (September 1995), pp. 551–597.

Manoguerra, A.S., "Toxic plant ingestion," *Emergency*, 23, no. 6 (June 1991), pp. 26–29.

_____ . "Poisonous plants: Part II," *Emergency*, 23, no. 7 (July 1991), pp. 23–26.

Myers, D.P., and Anderson, A.R., "Adolescent addiction: Assessment and identification," *Journal of Pediatric Health Care*, 5, no. 2 (March/April 1991), pp. 86–93.

Tenebein, M., "General management principles for poisoning." In Barkin, R.M., ed., *Pediatric Emergency Medicine: Concepts and Clinical Practice*. St. Louis: Mosby Year Book, Inc., 1992, pp. 463–470.

Washburn, P., "Identification, assessment, and referral of adolescent drug abusers," *Pediatric Nursing*, 17, no. 2 (March/April, 1991) pp. 137–140.

Pediatric Trauma Assessment

OBJECTIVES

When you have completed this chapter you should be able to

▶ List the most common causes of trauma to the child and the most frequent injuries to the child with multiple trauma.
▶ Describe the steps of the initial assessment.
▶ Describe effective airway management and ventilation in an injured child.
▶ List signs that may indicate hypoperfusion (shock) in the child.
▶ Describe management of the injured child in hypoperfusion (shock).
▶ Describe the essential components of the focused history and detailed physical exam.

Introduction

Trauma is the leading cause of death in children in the United States today. Statistics show that half of all childhood fatalities, approximately 6700 children under 15 years of age, occur each year as a result of injury. Motor vehicle crashes are the mechanism of injury in 40% of cases; this is followed by drowning, burns, falls, and firearms. Pediatric patients make up 10% to 15% of trauma seen in the emergency setting and are nearly twice as likely as adults to die in transport to the hospital or during resuscitation in the emergency department.

Mechanism of Injury

Even though children's tissues (muscles, blood vessels, bone, organs) have great elasticity and an ability to resume their original shape after being stretched, those tissues cannot withstand damage from forces such as inward pressure, excess stretching, or squeezing. Children also experience shearing type injuries caused when one part of the body slides over an adjacent part, such as occurs in major head injuries when the base of the brain slides over the bony ridges of the floor of the skull.

A child with a severe chest injury may not have any rib fractures because of the pliability of the rib cage, but the energy transmitted through the chest wall can cause major damage to the lungs, heart, and great blood vessels. Because of the mobility of organs within the chest, tension pneumothorax is a potentially life-threatening disorder. (See Chapter 11, "Chest, Abdominal, and Extremity Injuries.") Lap belts designed to prevent ejections from automobiles may leave only a small bruise on the abdomen, but the energy transmitted through the abdomen may cause liver or spleen lacerations, intestinal perforations, or even a spinal cord injury.

While falls are the most common injury in children, they cause fewer deaths because injuries are generally less severe. Even though penetrating injuries are less common in younger children, but increasing among adolescents, they are responsible for the highest death rate. The incidence of penetrating trauma is associated with the availability of weapons in and out of the home, especially in urban environments. Blunt trauma, accounting for approximately 90% of all pediatric trauma, is the most common cause of childhood trauma.

The most common childhood injuries seen in multiple trauma resulting from a motor vehicle crash affect the head, trunk, and extremity (triad of injury). It is not unusual for a child hit by a vehicle to sustain a head injury, lung contusion, spleen laceration, and femur fracture (Figure 9.1).

FIGURE 9.1
The triad of injury associated with a child pedestrian-motor vehicle crash includes injury to the head, chest, and femur.

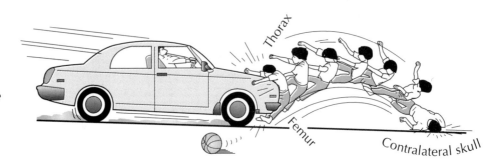

Initial Assessment

The sequence of pediatric assessment and management at the scene is similar to the care of the injured adult—immediately recognize and treat life-threatening conditions.

Airway

Assessment

When approaching the child, first check the airway. If the child is talking, crying, or answering questions, the child's airway is adequate and patent *at this time.* Because the child's airway is smaller in diameter than an adult's, it can be easily obstructed by blood, vomitus, tongue, and broken teeth. During the initial and detailed trauma assessment, reevaluate the airway frequently because respiratory compromise can occur, especially if there is an underlying head injury. Repeated assessment will alert you to the need for any advanced procedures to maintain the airway.

CAUTION!

With any head injury or other major injury, assume cervical spine injury. A fracture can only be ruled out by X ray at the receiving hospital.

Look for spontaneous chest motion and listen for spontaneous breath sounds, diminished breath sounds, or other sounds such as stridor, bubbling, or gurgling (Figure 9.2).

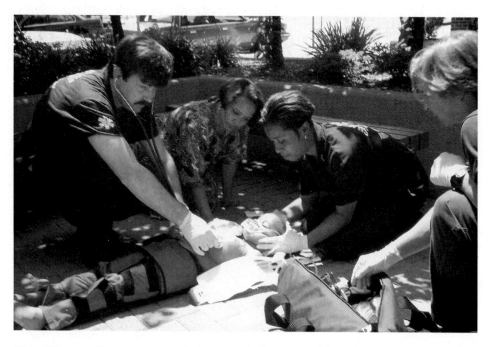

FIGURE 9.2   *Reassessment of airway, ventilation, and breath sounds while maintaining cervical spine stabilization.*

Management

BLS providers should provide the following care in cases of an obstructed airway:

- Control and stabilize the C-spine in neutral alignment.
- Place the child in neutral or "sniffing" position and perform the jaw-thrust maneuver to bring the tongue even further forward in the mouth.
- Suction the mouth to remove mucus, blood, or vomitus. Head-injured children are at risk for posttraumatic seizures and vomiting.
- Provide oxygen to the child before using airway adjuncts to establish or maintain the airway.
- Insert an oral airway carefully in the unconscious child if necessary. (See Chapter 4, "Equipment and Procedures for Management of ABCs.")
- Administer high-flow, high-concentration oxygen when the airway is secured.

ALS providers should consider the following additional care for airway management:

- Endotracheal intubation should be performed when the airway remains inadequate or airway control must be secured to free the provider for other tasks. Recheck the placement of the tube frequently because minimal movement may displace it (Figure 9.3).
- Needle cricothyrotomy is indicated only in the rare instance of severe facial trauma or unresolved upper airway obstruction. It is a last-ditch effort to establish an airway.

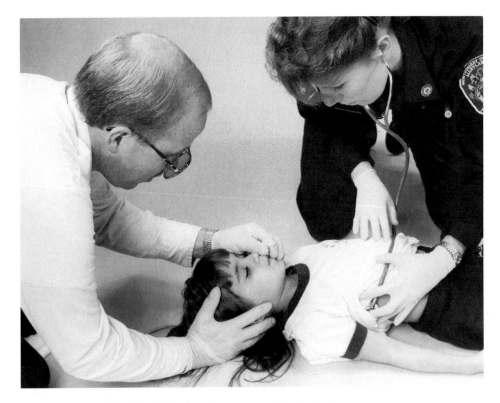

FIGURE 9.3 *Checking ET tube placement prior to taping.*

Breathing

Assessment

Observe the child's color. Check for pallor, mottling, or cyanosis of the lips, tongue, mucous membranes of the mouth, and nail beds.

Assess breathing with the child's chest and abdomen exposed. To count the respiratory rate in young children, observe the rise and fall of the abdomen. Remember the expected respiratory rate of the child. Rates lower than 20 breaths/min in a small child may indicate ventilatory failure due to chest muscle fatigue. Rates greater than 60/min indicate oxygen hunger, reflective of ineffective breathing.

Inspect the chest, noting any swelling or bruising or penetrating chest wounds. Look for other irregularities such as retractions, unequal rise and fall of the chest, use of accessory muscles of the chest wall, paradoxical breathing or "see-sawing" of the chest and abdomen. Note other signs of respiratory distress such as nasal flaring, apprehension, noisy breathing, or hoarseness. Decreased responsiveness can also be a sign of hypoxia.

Using a stethoscope, listen for bilateral breath sounds under each clavicle and at the midaxillary line halfway between the axilla and the lower margin of the rib cage. Note any wheezing or other abnormalities such as unequal or diminished breath sounds.

Palpate for tracheal deviation, which is a sign of tension pneumothorax. This is especially difficult to evaluate in young children, owing to their short, chubby necks; thus, *DO NOT* rely on this as the only sign of a tension pneumothorax.

Management

BLS providers should administer the following intervention for children in acute respiratory distress or failure:

- Monitor ABCs and vital signs.
- Administer high-flow, high-concentration oxygen.
- Perform mouth-to-mask ventilation until positive pressure ventilation can be implemented.
- Provide positive pressure ventilation when the respiratory rate is less than 20 breaths/min or the child is not breathing. NOTE: The mask must be the correct size and fit to achieve effective ventilations.
- Treat open chest wounds immediately with a petroleum gauze dressing or cellophane taped on three corners of the gauze. Monitor the ABCs and burp the dressing to release pressure if a tension pneumothorax develops (Figure 9.4).
- Administer CPR if necessary.
- Transport patient *immediately*.

ALS providers should additionally provide the following management for life-threatening ventilation problems:

- Endotracheal intubation.
- If tension pneumothorax develops, perform needle thoracostomy to relieve the intrathoracic pressure.

Circulation

The child's blood volume is proportional to weight (Table 3.2). A 3-year-old child with a total blood volume of 1275 ml will be in hypoperfusion (shock) with a loss of 255 ml of blood (about 1 cup). Young children may develop significant hypovolemic shock from a scalp laceration (Figure 9.5).

Initial Assessment

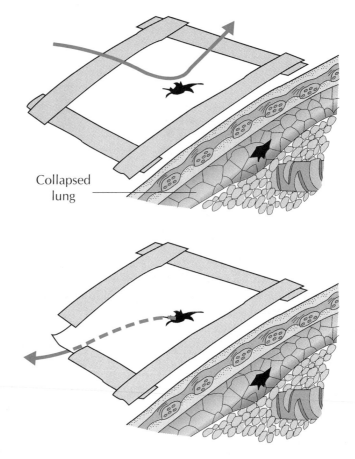

FIGURE 9.4 *Management of sucking chest wound. Cover an open chest wound with cellophane or petroleum gauze dressing taped on three corners of the gauze to prevent air entry on inspiration. Peel back a corner of the dressing if tension pneumothorax occurs to permit air escape on expiration.*

Collapsed lung

Identification of *early hypoperfusion (shock)* is extremely important in children because of their physiologic ability to compensate for shock. As shock develops, they will constrict their arteries and veins, actually shunting blood to the central circulation. As blood loss increases, this compensatory mechanism becomes less effective. Once the blood pressure begins dropping, usually after 25% blood loss, the child is in *late* shock. Resuscitation of the child in late shock is more difficult because the condition will deteriorate very rapidly (Table 9.1).

FIGURE 9.5 *Applying manual pressure to scalp laceration to control bleeding.*

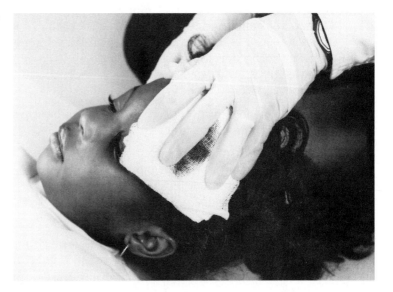

TABLE 9.1 ■ *Systemic Responses to Hemorrhage in the Pediatric Patient*

Body System	Early (< 25% blood volume loss)	Prehypotensive (25% blood volume loss)	Hypotensive (40% blood volume loss)
Circulatory	Increased heart rate; weak thready pulse	Increased heart rate, thready pulse	Decreased systolic BP, tachycardia to bradycardia
Nervous	Normal, anxious, irritable, combative	Confused, decreased responsiveness, dulled response to pain	Unconscious
Skin	Cool, clammy	Cyanotic, decreased capillary refill, cold extremities	Pale, cold

Source: Adapted from: Waisman, Y., and Eichelberger, M.R., "Hypovolemic Shock." In Eichelberger, M.R., ed., *Pediatric Trauma: Prevention, Acute Care, Rehabilitation.* St. Louis: Mosby Year Book, 1993, p. 182.

Assessment

Assess the patient's circulation by observing the child's color. Look for any obvious bleeding and investigate any dark stains on clothing. Apply direct pressure and elevation to control bleeding. Check the capillary refill time. Because of the child's tendency to become hypothermic, perform this test in an area of central circulation, such as over the forehead or sternum. A capillary refill time longer than 2 seconds indicates poor perfusion.

Auscultate the chest, listening for the apical heart rate below and medial to the left nipple. Because of the child's thin chest wall, the heart sounds should be clear and distinct. Note any muffling or indistinct sounds of the heart that might indicate cardiac tamponade. Palpate the pulse rate and check for weak or absent brachial or femoral pulses. Take the blood pressure.

The best indicators of *early hypoperfusion (shock)* in children are:

■ Sustained tachycardia (greater than 130 beats/min) in a quiet child;
■ Increased capillary refill time greater than 2 seconds;
■ Cool, pale skin.

Altered mental status is also associated with hypoperfusion (shock); however, this sign may be difficult to evaluate when head trauma is suspected.

A drop in the systolic blood pressure is a late indicator of hypoperfusion (shock). The child will have lost at least 25% of the total blood volume before a decrease in systolic blood pressure is noted. The child with a systolic blood pressure less than 70 mm Hg is in late shock. If a child shows signs and symptoms of shock without obvious hemorrhage be suspicious of internal bleeding. The body spaces of the chest, abdomen, and pelvis can harbor large enough quantities of blood to put a child into shock. Except for small infants, bleeding into the skull alone does not cause shock; it causes increased intracranial pressure.

Children with hypothermia also have a delayed capillary refill time and cool, mottled, or pale extremities. Their pulse rate and blood pressure will usually be within normal limits or low. The child with altered mental status and cool, pale skin who has a capillary refill time of 2 seconds or less and a systolic blood pressure of 100 may have a head injury or other central nervous system dysfunction rather than hypovolemic shock.

Management

BLS providers should provide the following care to children with life-threatening circulatory problems:

- Control external bleeding by placing a dressing with direct pressure over the site and elevate the extremity if indicated. Use your entire hand to place direct pressure on a scalp laceration, in case there is a skull fracture underneath. Manual pressure is better than a "pressure dressing."
- Place pressure over a pulse point between the heart and the bleeding site to control a bleeding artery. Use the brachial artery in the upper extremity and use the femoral artery in the lower extremity.
- Administer high-flow, high-concentration oxygen by nonrebreather mask.
- Keep the child warm.
- Apply PASG for pelvic fractures if protocols so direct and an appropriate size is available. (See Chapter 4, "Equipment and Procedures for Management of ABCs," and Figure 4.22 for indications and application directions.) *Transparent* pneumatic splints may be used to control bleeding and fractures.
- Transport patient *immediately.*

ALS providers should additionally perform the following management as directed by medical direction or protocols:

- Start an IV with Ringer's Lactate or Normal Saline. *DO NOT* delay transport to start the IV. Limit your attempts to two sticks en route to the hospital. If the extrication is lengthy, attempt IV start at the scene.
- If the child is unconscious and in severe hypovolemic shock, and attempts at a peripheral line are unsuccessful, insert an IO line if local protocols permit.
- Administer a fluid bolus (20 ml/kg), as rapidly as possible, IV push with a syringe or pressure bag. Use warm fluids if possible.
- Recheck the child's vital signs and capillary refill for signs of improved circulatory perfusion. If signs of shock do not improve after 5 minutes, repeat the fluid bolus. Up to three boluses may be needed in severe shock.
- Transport patient *immediately.*

Disability: Neurologic Exam

A decreased level of responsiveness commonly results from hypoxia, hypovolemia, or a head injury. No improvement with oxygenation, or progressive deterioration, indicates either a massive injury or that complications of the injury have occurred.

Assessment

Initial assessment of the neurologic status of a child is made using *AVPU* to describe the child's level of responsiveness—**A**lert, responsive to **V**erbal stimuli, responsive to **P**ainful stimuli, or **U**nresponsive. The Glasgow Coma Scale (GCS) provides a standardized, quantifiable evaluation of neurologic status. It can be repeated over time by prehospital and hospital personnel to determine whether the child is improving or deteriorating. Documentation is important in order to monitor the trend in neurologic status over time. (See Table 3.4 for GCS criteria.) Palpate the skull for obvious fractures or deformities. Observe for decorticate or decerebrate posturing.

Management

The BLS provider should provide the following care if altered mental status is present and head injury is suspected:

- Administer high-flow, high-concentration oxygen by bag-valve mask.
- If head injury is suspected, hyperventilate at a rate of 5 to 10 breaths faster than the child's normal respiratory rate.
- Elevate the head and upper body as a unit, unless contraindicated, maintaining immobilization of the spine.
- Observe and prepare for posttraumatic seizure.

ALS providers should start an IV if the child demonstrates signs of hypovolemic shock.

Exposure

Before removing the child's clothes, remember that children have a tendency to develop hypothermia. Infants and children cool more quickly than do adults, even in mild weather, because of their greater body surface area to mass ratio. Children with hypothermia (core body temperature less than 98°F) do not respond as well to resuscitation efforts. Drug absorption will also be delayed.

Assessment

Expose only that body part being assessed to reduce heat loss. Once assessment of that body part is completed, recover it and move on to another body part. Observe the child for signs of mild hypothermia, such as cool, pale, or mottled extremities and an increased capillary refill time greater than 2 seconds in the extremities.

Management

All prehospital providers should provide the following care to the child with potential for heat loss:

- Cover the child to retain body heat during further assessment, management, and transport. Also cover the head of infants and children.
- Use warmed oxygen and IV fluids, if possible, during cold weather. Turn the ambulance heater on.

Focused History and Detailed Physical Exam

When the ABCDEs of the initial assessment are under control, proceed to the focused history and detailed physical exam. Transport immediately if your initial assessment reveals life-threatening injuries, respiratory distress, or hypoperfusion (shock). In this circumstance, the focused history and detailed physical exam is done in the back of the ambulance. Do not delay transport for treating wounds or applying traction at the scene if the child's survival is in danger. Remember to reassess the ABCDEs frequently during care.

Minimal time should be spent in the field with the focused history and detailed physical exam. In many cases, the physical exam is performed during transport. A rapid trauma assessment is performed in a systematic order to find additional injuries and plan management strategies during transport. Use the same systematic approach as you assess each part of the body. Check for the following: deformities, contusions (bruises), abrasions, penetrations, burns, tenderness, lacerations, and swelling. For example, bruises on the abdomen will alert you to the possibility of internal bleeding and the potential for the child to develop hypoperfusion (shock).

While some of the child's history has been obtained during the initial assessment, complete information about the child's history using the SAMPLE format, including allergies, medications taken, past medical history, last oral intake, and events surrounding the occurrence of the injury. In addition, gather further information about the mechanism of injury from family members or bystanders.

Head and Neck

- Palpate the head for any lacerations, swelling, deformities, or depressions.
- Check eye movement for coordination in following objects and note if the eyes are focusing. Use a penlight to check pupils for size, shape, and reaction to light.
- Look for any blood or fluid drainage in the ears, nose, and mouth. Any bruising around the eyes (raccoon sign) or behind the ears (Battle's sign) are both late signs of basilar skull fracture. Clear fluid draining from the nose may indicate a basilar fracture in the cribriform plate of the nose.
- Palpate the facial structure and neck for any swelling, deformity, or depression (Figure 9.6). Check for proper alignment of the mandible and any missing teeth. Complaint of pain on palpation of the neck is an important sign of neck injury in children.
- Palpate the infant's fontanelle for tense bulging (may indicate increased intracranial pressure). A depressed fontanelle indicates hypovolemia.

FIGURE 9.6 *Palpate for facial deformity.*

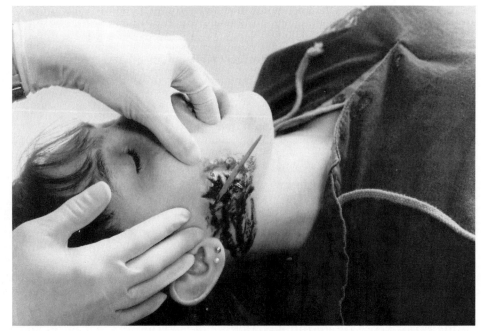

Chapter 9: Pediatric Trauma Assessment

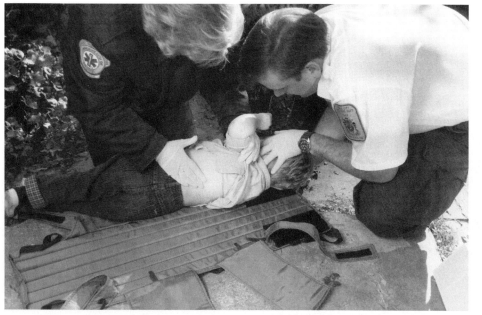

FIGURE 9.7 As you logroll the child onto a backboard, quickly inspect and palpate the back and spine.

Back

As you logroll the child to place him or her on the backboard, quickly inspect and palpate the patient's back, spine, and buttocks. Note any deformities, contusions, abrasions, penetrations, burns, tenderness, lacerations, and swelling (Figure 9.7).

Chest

This exam should have been completed during the initial assessment.

Abdomen

- Lightly palpate the abdomen, noting any guarding, tenderness, pain, or rigidity (Figure 9.8).
- Inspect for deformities, contusions, abrasions, penetrations, burns, tenderness, lacerations, and swelling.
- Check the femoral area, noting any swelling or hematomas and presence of pulses.
- Palpate pelvic girdle for tenderness or deformity. Carefully compress the pelvis by pushing the two wings of the ilium toward the symphysis pubis to determine if this maneuver is painful, indicating a pelvic fracture.
- Inspect genitalia and perineal areas for hematoma. Blood at the urethra and ecchymosis of the perineum may indicate bladder rupture or pelvic fracture.

Extremities

- Manually examine the arms and legs, noting obvious deformity, swelling, and open wounds with or without exposed bone.
- Assess vascular status distal to the injury by checking for the presence of a pulse, color and temperature of the extremity, and capillary refill time.

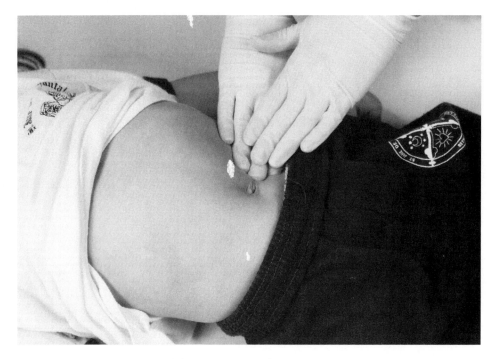

FIGURE 9.8 *Palpate the abdomen for guarding, pain, tenderness, and rigidity.*

- Note any loss of sensation, pain, or tenderness on palpation or motion; inability to move the extremity; asymmetry of extremities or improper alignment. Note excessive pain that persists after immobilization. This could indicate *compartment syndrome,* a condition in which the pressure within the closed space of a muscle increases to the point where the blood supply is inadequate to oxygenate tissue. The pressure might be caused by hemorrhage, swelling of tissues, or a tight tourniquet like dressing. It is extremely painful and requires emergency surgical intervention at the hospital.
- Palpate all major joints and long bones. Significant swelling can arise from displacement, which can also lead to nerve and blood vessel damage.
- Periodically check and recheck pulse and capillary refill distal to the injured extremity (Figures 9.9 and 3.12).

FIGURE 9.9
Assessing capillary refill time.

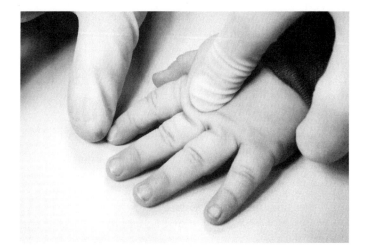

Chapter 9: Pediatric Trauma Assessment

Management

All prehospital providers should continue assessment and management of the ABCDEs and transport the child.

■ For orthopedic injuries to the upper extremities, splint the extremity in the position in which it was found. If there is no pulse present, realign and splint.

■ For injury to the lower extremities between the hip and knee, apply gentle traction in the line of the extremity and splint. Palpate for the presence of a distal pulse before and after realignment and after splinting.

■ Cover any open wounds near a fracture site with a sterile dressing. Be sure to report any suspicion of an open fracture to the emergency department.

For more information about specific chest, abdominal, and extremity injuries, refer to Chapter 11, "Chest, Abdominal, and Extremity Injuries."

Pediatric Trauma Assessment References

Chamberlain, J.M., "Algorithm for pediatric trauma." In Eichelberger, M.R., *Pediatric Trauma: Prevention, Acute Care, Rehabilitation.* St. Louis: Mosby Year Book, Inc., 1993.

Cox, D.M., "Trauma fluid resuscitation," *Emergency, 26,* no. 4 (April 1994), pp. 22–26.

Crosby, L.A., and Lewaller, D.G., *Emergency Care and Transportation of the Sick and Injured.* Rosemont, IL: American Academy of Orthopedic Surgeons, 1995.

Eichelberger, M.R., and Anderson, K.D., "Sequelae of thoracic injury in children." In Hix, W.R., and Aaron, B.L., eds., *Residua of Thoracic Trauma.* Mount Kisco, NY: Futura Publishing Co., 1987, pp. 247–264.

Glaeser, P.W., and Losek, J.D., "Emergency intraosseous infusions in children," *American Journal of Emergency Medicine,* 4 (1986), p. 34.

Jones, W.T., "When your patient gets shocky: Managing hypovolemia," *JEMS,* 17, no. 7 (July 1992), pp. 48–53.

McSwain, N.E., "PASG in the '90s," *Emergency, 26,* no. 4 (April 1994) pp. 28–33.

Peclet, M.H., Newman, K.D., Eichelberger, M.R., et al., "Patterns of injury in children," *Journal of Pediatric Surgery,* 22, (1990), pp. 85–91.

Rimar, J.M., "Shock in infants and children: Assessment and treatment," *Maternal and Child Nursing,* 13, (March/April 1988), pp. 98–105.

Shoor, P.M., Berryhill, R.E., and Benumof, J.L., "Intraosseous infusion: Pressure flow relationship and pharmacokinetics," *Journal of Trauma,* 19 (1979) p. 772.

Spivey, W.H., "Intraosseous infusions," *Journal of Pediatrics,* 111 (1987), p. 639.

Young G.M., Eichelberger, M.R., "Initial resuscitation of the child with multiple injuries." In Grossman, M., Dickmann, R.A., eds., *Pediatric Emergency Medicine: A Clinician's Reference.* Philadelphia: Lippincott, 1990.

Head and Spinal Cord Injury

OBJECTIVES

When you have completed this chapter you should be able to

▶ List and describe the types of skull fractures.
▶ List and describe the types of injuries to the brain.
▶ List the characteristics of head injury.
▶ Describe the assessment and management of the head-injured child.
▶ Describe the assessment and management of the spinal cord injury.

Head Injury

Head injury claims the lives of 10 out of every 100,000 American children between 1 and 14 years of age annually. Death or disability from head injury affects the lives of 25,000 children each year. Up to 75% of all children sustaining multiple trauma suffer head injury, and nearly 80% of all trauma deaths in children are associated with significant neurologic injury.

The mechanism of head trauma varies by age and development abilities of the child and his or her environmental exposure to these mechanisms.

- Infants and small children most commonly fall, either off the bed, out of the crib, down a flight of stairs, or out of windows.
- Children frequently sustain head injuries from bicycle and skateboard accidents, rollerblading, horseback riding, climbing trees, etc.
- Older children and adolescents sustain head injuries from sports injuries, such as soccer, football, and diving.
- Motor vehicle crashes involving unrestrained passengers and pedestrians also account for many serious head injuries.
- Penetrating trauma is seen in suicide or homicide cases primarily in the adolescent.
- Child abuse occurs at any age. Shaken-baby syndrome is a frequent cause of head injury in abused infants. The infant is shaken so hard that the bridging veins in the head rupture and cause a subdural hematoma. (See Chapter 13, "Child Abuse.")

Anatomy and Physiology

Children are particularly susceptible to head injury because their heads are proportionately larger and heavier in comparison to the rest of their body. In addition, the musculoskeletal structures of the neck are not as strong as an adult's, making the child more susceptible to high cervical spine injuries. Because a child's head is so large, a significantly larger blood flow goes to the head and brain. The scalp is highly vascular. Children can bleed enough from a scalp laceration to develop shock if not properly treated. The cranial bones are also thinner and less developed, thus being more susceptible to brain injury.

The skull is an enclosed space containing brain tissue, cerebrospinal fluid, and blood, all of which function in balance. When the brain swells or hemorrhage occurs within this confined space, it places pressure on brain tissue, compressing arteries and veins, which cuts off the oxygen supply and other nutrients to the brain. The brain's protective response is to call for more blood, which is one cause of diffuse cerebral edema.

Increased intracranial pressure (ICP) due to diffuse cerebral edema is common in children. It generally occurs slowly over several hours or days following the initial injury. Seizures and vomiting may occur after the intracranial pressure level has begun to increase.

Increased intracranial pressure, if untreated, is fatal because of increased pressure on the respiratory center of the brain. However, intracranial pressure is better tolerated for a short time in infants than adults because the skull sutures are not fused and the anterior fontanelle allows expansion of the skull to accommodate the bleeding or swollen tissue.

Because of the rapid maturation of the brain, which occurs between 2 and 8 years of age, the skull and brain of children over 8 years of age respond to trauma similar to that of an adult.

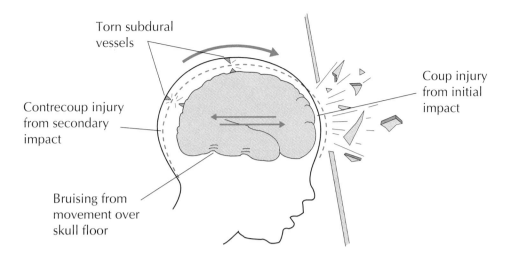

Torn subdural vessels

Contrecoup injury from secondary impact

Coup injury from initial impact

Bruising from movement over skull floor

FIGURE 10.1 *Coup and contrecoup injury: note movement and bruising of the frontal area of the brain at time of initial impact—stretching brain tissue, tearing subdural vessels, and bruising, as the brain moves over the floor of the skull. The occipital (posterior) area of the brain is bruised as the brain bounces back to strike the back of the skull.*

Mechanism of Injury

The brain of infants and young children is less myelinated, and the tissue is thinner, more fragile, and easily bruised. With an acceleration-deceleration injury, the brain receives a *coup and contrecoup* injury (Figure 10.1). For example, if the child falls and hits the back of the head, the back part of the brain impacts the skull at the injury site and then the frontal lobes of the brain hit the skull opposite the injury site. This brain movement within the skull results in shearing and tearing of small blood vessels, as the brain is jolted back and forth.

Types of Head Injury

Fractures

A *linear* skull fracture occurs along one of the skull's suture lines. A fracture across the temporal bone may tear the middle meningeal artery, resulting in an epidural hemorrhage.

A *depressed* skull fracture is palpable on physical examination, usually 5 mm below the contour of the skull. The brain tissue underneath may be contused or lacerated.

A *compound* skull fracture is an open fracture, either linear or depressed, under a scalp laceration (Figure 10.2).

A *basilar* skull fracture is a fracture on the floor of the skull. Leakage of clear or amber-colored cerebrospinal fluid from the nose or ear indicates a cribriform plate fracture inside the skull. Other signs of a basilar skull fracture include bruising under the eyes (raccoon eyes) or behind the ear (Battle's sign).

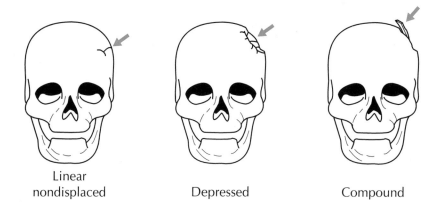

FIGURE 10.2 *Skull fractures.*

Linear
nondisplaced   Depressed   Compound

Concussion

This is a violent shaking or jarring of the brain that results in transient loss of consciousness disappearing within either minutes or days. There is no permanent neurologic damage. Other symptoms may include headache, vomiting, and memory loss or confusion. The child is usually not hospitalized unless loss of consciousness lasts longer than 5 minutes or persistent vomiting is present (Figure 10.3A).

Contusion

Scalp, forehead, or *facial* contusions are associated with local swelling and tenderness with variable bruising. There is usually no neurological deficit.

Brain contusions represent a severe injury with hemorrhage and swelling in the brain tissue, usually resulting in marked alterations in level of consciousness (Figure 10.3B). Other symptoms may include a disturbance in strength or sensation, seizures, or a change in visual awareness.

Hemorrhage

An *epidural* hemorrhage occurs with a skull fracture and meningeal artery bleed located between the skull and the dura. A *subdural* hematoma results from a laceration of the vein network between the dura and the surface of the brain. These hematomas can occur hours to days after the injury. An *intracerebral* hemorrhage results from a brain laceration (Figure 10.4).

Patient Care

History

During assessment it is important to note the mechanism of injury and establish by history the circumstances surrounding the injury. The following information should be obtained from parents, teachers, or bystanders:

S   Did the child have a seizure before or after the head injury? Did the child vomit? If so, how long after the head injury? Was the child less responsive or lose consciousness immediately after the injury or at a later time? Was the child ever disoriented after the head injury? How long did the loss of consciousness or disorientation last? If the child can answer questions, are there any visual disturbances, headache, or tingling or numbness in the extremities?

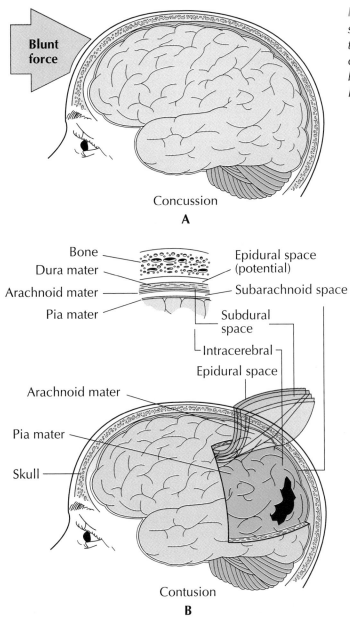

FIGURE 10.3 (A) Concussion vs. (B) contusion. Closed head injuries: (A) In a concussion, there is no detectable brain damage. (B) In a contusion, there is bruising or rupturing of the brain tissue and vessels at any of the identified levels.

Concussion

A

Bone
Dura mater
Arachnoid mater
Pia mater

Epidural space (potential)
Subarachnoid space
Subdural space
Intracerebral
Epidural space

Arachnoid mater

Pia mater

Skull

Contusion

B

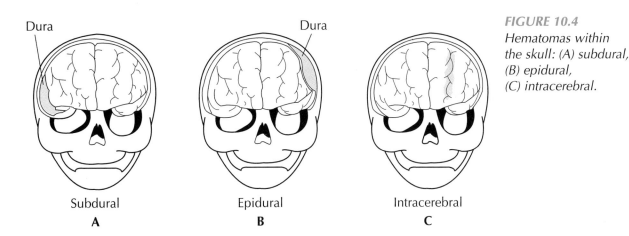

FIGURE 10.4
Hematomas within the skull: (A) subdural, (B) epidural, (C) intracerebral.

Dura

Dura

Subdural

A

Epidural

B

Intracerebral

C

A   Does the child have any allergies?

M   Does the child take any medications?

P   Does the child have a history of seizures? Does the child have any other health problems or chronic illnesses?

L   When was the child's last oral intake? What was it?

E   What happened? Was the child struck on the head or did the child fall? What was the height of the fall? What was the approximate force of the injury? When did the injury occur?

Assessment

Expect any child with a head injury to have an associated cervical spine injury. Some children will have a maxillofacial injury, so carefully inspect the airway for teeth, blood, mucus, and loss of continuity of the jaw when performing the initial trauma assessment.

After assessment and management of the ABCs, assess the level of consciousness with the Glasgow Coma Scale (Table 3.4). Ask older children questions to test their orientation to time, place, and person. Altered mental status is present when a child asks the same question over and over, even when it has already been answered. Combativeness can be a sign of hypoxia or hypoperfusion (shock).

The child with a head injury may be alert or have any level of alteration in level of consciousness: lethargy, stupor, or coma. Note any decorticate, decerebrate, or other abnormal posturing in the comatose child.

Detailed Physical Exam

Inspect and palpate the skull for fractures or depressions. Note any clear or amber drainage from the nose or ears, which is indicative of a basilar skull fracture. Check for bruising behind the ear (Battle's sign) or around the eyes (raccoon eyes), signaling a basilar skull fracture.

Check pupillary response, noting size of the pupils and their reactivity to bright light. Asymmetry of pupil size, abnormal lateral gaze, and roving eye movements are indications of head trauma (Figure 10.5). (See Table 10.1 for characteristics associated with mild, moderate, and severe head injuries.)

CAUTION!

SHOCK IN CHILDREN WITH HEAD INJURY

Children with signs of hypovolemic shock (hypoperfusion) generally have other associated injuries. Only infants who have an open fontanelle and open sutures can hold enough blood in the head to cause hypovolemic shock. If there is an associated cervical spine injury, the child may be in *neurogenic* shock. Signs of hypovolemic shock include tachycardia and cool, clammy skin. In contrast, signs of neurogenic shock include bradycardia and warm, dry extremities.

Increased Intracranial Pressure

In the early stages of rising intracranial pressure (ICP), the blood pressure may be elevated, the heart rate is slow, and breathing is slow and deep, alternating with rapid deep breaths (Cheyne-Stokes respiration). The child

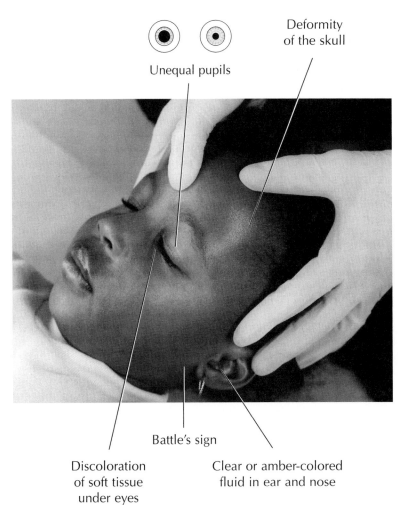

Unequal pupils

Deformity of the skull

FIGURE 10.5 *Inspect the skull and head for signs of a skull fracture.*

Battle's sign

Discoloration of soft tissue under eyes

Clear or amber-colored fluid in ear and nose

TABLE 10.1 ■ *Characteristics of Head Injury with Varying Severity*

CHARACTERISTIC	MILD	MODERATE	SEVERE
Consciousness	Transient loss Altered mental status	Loss of consciousness	Coma
Glasgow Coma Score	14–15	9–13	< 9
Behavior	Crying, agitated, easily consoled	Agitated, combative, not easily consoled	Quiet, unresponsive
Signs	Local tissue swelling Redness over injury site	Moves spontaneously May have CSF leak Pupils reactive	Bulging fontanelle Pupils unresponsive Posturing Increased intracranial pressure (ICP)
Type of Injury	Simple skull fracture Concussion	Hemorrhage (subdural, epidural, intraventricular)	Brain laceration Acute subdural and intracerebral hematoma

Source: Developed by author.

is responsive to pain and might demonstrate decorticate posturing. Typical decorticate posturing includes adduction of the arms at the shoulders; the arms are flexed on the chest with the wrists flexed and the hands fisted; and the lower extremities are extended and adducted.

The infant with ICP has a bulging fontanelle, irritability, and listlessness. The child usually exhibits altered mental status along with the three signs of the Cushing's reflex (widening pulse pressure, decreasing heart rate, and abnormal respirations). As the intracranial pressure continues to rise, the systolic blood pressure increases while the heart and respiratory rates decrease. Pupils become fixed and dilated, and the child becomes flaccid and unresponsive to pain. This child needs immediate transport and efficient prehospital management.

The findings at the scene, on reassessment during transport, and how they change over time are essential to detect signs of deterioration or improvement in the child. This information is important for the receiving hospital to plan definitive treatment of the head-injured child.

Management

Effective recognition of the head-injured child with hypoxia and hypovolemia along with aggressive intervention can save a child's life and prevent secondary brain injury and long-term disability.

BLS field care of the child with a head injury should include the following:

- Assess and monitor the ABCs and neurologic status.
- In the case of a facial injury, suction blood, mucus, and vomitus from patient's airway. Remove broken teeth. *DO NOT insert a nasogastric tube or suction catheter in the nose if a cerebrospinal fluid leak, raccoon eyes, or Battle's sign are present.*
- Maintain the airway in the unconscious child by jaw-thrust or insert an oral airway, using extreme care. The nasopharyngeal airway should not be used in the head-injured patient.
- Stabilize and immobilize the cervical spine.
- Using a bag-valve mask, hyperventilate the child with high-flow, high-concentration oxygen at a rate at least 5 breaths/min faster than the child's usual respiratory rate. This will increase the blood oxygen level and decrease the blood carbon dioxide level, causing constriction of the blood vessels. **This is the most effective method for temporarily lowering increased intracranial pressure.**
- Manage shock with PASG application if protocols permit. Hypovolemia must be managed even when increased intracranial pressure is present to allow adequate perfusion of brain tissue.
- Be alert for vomiting. Have suction ready.
- Cover any scalp lacerations and apply pressure to stop the bleeding. (See Chapter 9, "Pediatric Trauma Assessment.") Use your entire hand to apply pressure over an area of suspected skull fracture.
- Apply Normal Saline-soaked gauze to open fractures.
- *DO NOT* remove impaled foreign bodies.
- Cover injured eyes with a sterile gauze patch.
- Immediately transport patient.

ALS providers should also initiate the following additional care:

- Intubation to maintain the airway, only if necessary, such as in cases of long transport time or deteriorating respiratory status. (See "Intubation Risks" in box below.)

- Insert an IV of Ringer's Lactate or Normal Saline to run at a keep-open rate. In cases of hypovolemic shock, treat the child with boluses of Ringer's Lactate at 20 ml/kg IV push.

INTUBATION RISKS   *CAUTION!*

Intubation of the head-injured child is often difficult because of the need to keep the patient's neck stabilized. It also creates more risk for the child with facial or basilar skull fractures or increased intracranial pressure. In the case of the head-injured child, intubation in the controlled hospital setting is preferable to attempts in the field. Children can usually be adequately ventilated by bag-mask ventilation.

Spinal Cord Injury

Spinal cord injuries are fortunately not as common in children as they are in adults; however, the types of injuries that do occur in children are potentially life-threatening or may cause permanent disabilities. Major causes of spinal cord injuries in children are falls, motor vehicle crashes, and sports injuries. Cervical spine injuries occur in approximately 1% of all injured children; however, about 18% of children injured in a motor vehicle crash have an injury to the cervical spine.

Cervical Spine

By 8 years of age, the bony structure of the child's cervical spine has achieved an adult appearance on X ray. In the younger child, significant physiologic differences exist in the development of the spinal column that contribute to significant injuries.

- There is much greater mobility in the cervical spine of a young child because the vertebrae are wedge-shaped. Subluxation can occur with relatively little force.
- The fulcrum of neck motion occurs much higher in children (C2–3 level) than in adults (C5–6 level), leading to higher cervical spine injuries. The most common sites of cervical spine injury in young children are at C1, C2, and C3.
- Because the head is heavier, greater stress is placed on the spinal cord with flexion-extension injuries. The spinal cord is also less elastic than the ligaments and cartilage that protect it.
- The neck muscles of the infant are not well developed; some of the forces involved in injury are not reduced. Infants who have not yet achieved head control are at great risk for cervical spine injury.

Assessment

As with adults, assume there has been a cervical spine injury every time a head injury is suspected in the pediatric patient. During the detailed physical exam, assess for spontaneous and purposeful movement and sensation in the extremities. Pain on palpation of the neck is another sign of neck injury.

Management

All prehospital providers should institute immediate stabilization of the cervical spine while performing the initial assessment. Immobilize the infant or small child on a backboard with a small towel or pad at the shoulders to maintain the cervical spine in straight alignment. This will compensate for the large occiput of the child's head, which would normally result in a flexion of the cervical spine.

Lumbar Spine

The increased use of car safety seats has reduced the mortality from motor vehicle crashes. However, the advent of lap and shoulder restraints has increased certain types of injuries to the lumbar spine and abdominal organs in children. Lap belts are designed for placement below the anterior superior iliac spines. In children, the lap belts frequently position themselves across the abdomen because the pelvic bones are not fully developed. Spinal injury (dislocation, fracture, or subluxation of the vertebrae, or rupture of the spinal ligaments) is caused by hyperflexion of the spine around the lap belt (Figure 10.6). Abdominal injuries to the liver, spleen, bowel, bladder or mesentery occur because of compression and stretching of tissue. (See Chapter 11, "Chest, Abdominal, and Extremity Injuries," for a description of abdominal injuries.) For children who have outgrown the child safety seat, the lap and shoulder restraint combination usually results in less serious injuries. However, there can be fractures to the ribs, clavicle, sternum, and underlying organs of lungs, heart, and great vessels.

Assessment

During the detailed physical exam of any child passenger in a motor vehicle crash, ask the parent if the lap belt was fastened, and then inspect the abdomen for the classic sign of abdominal bruising and abrasion in the shape of the lap belt.

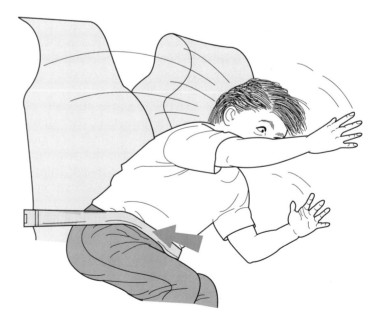

FIGURE 10.6   Forces on the abdomen and lumbar spine from a lap belt in cases of an accelerating-decelerating injury.

Chapter 10: Head and Spinal Cord Injury

Management

All prehospital providers should provide the following care to the child with a suspected lumbar spine injury from the lap-belt syndrome.

- Place the child on a backboard and immobilize the entire spine.
- Assess and manage any potential shock from the abdominal injuries as outlined in the sections in Chapter 9 dealing with the initial assessment and detailed physical exam.

Head and Spinal Cord Injury References

Arbour, R., "What you can do to reduce increased I.C.P.," *Nursing*, 93, (November 1993), pp. 41–46.

Dickman, C.A., and Rekate, H.L., "Spinal trauma." In Eichelberger, M.R., ed., *Pediatric Trauma: Prevention, Acute Care, Rehabilitation.* St. Louis: Mosby Year Book, Inc., 1993, pp. 362–377.

Dolan, M.A., "Head injury." In Barkin, R.M., ed., *Pediatric Emergency Medicine: Concepts and Clinical Practice.* St. Louis: Mosby Year Book, Inc., 1992, pp. 184–198.

Easton, A., "Respiratory involvement in pediatric head injury," *JEMS*, 18, no. 4 (April 1993), pp. 63–66.

Fuchs, S., et al., "Cervical spine fractures sustained by young children in forward-facing car seats," *Pediatrics*, 84, no. 2 (August 1989), pp. 348–354.

Glassman, E.S., Johnson, J.R., and Holt, R.T., "Seatbelt injuries in children," *Journal of Trauma*, 33 (1992), p. 822.

Herzenberg, J.E., and Hensinger, R.N., "Pediatric cervical spine injuries," *Trauma Quarterly*, 5, no. 2 (1989) p. 73.

Luerssen, T.G., "General characteristics of neurologic injury." In Eichelberger, M.R., ed., *Pediatric Trauma: Prevention, Acute Care, Rehabilitation.* St. Louis: Mosby Year Book, Inc., 1993, pp. 345–352.

Mayer, T., et al., "The modified injury severity scale in pediatric multiple trauma patients." *Journal of Pediatric Surgery*, 15, no. 6 (December 1980), pp. 719–726.

Newman, K.D., et al., "The lap belt complex: Intestinal and lumbar spine injury in children," *Journal of Trauma*, 30 (1990) pp. 1133–1140.

Patterson, R.J., Brown, G.W., Salassi-Scotter, M., and Middaugh, D., "Head injury in the conscious child," *American Journal of Nursing*, 92, no, 8 (August 1992), pp. 22–27.

Sivit, C.J., et al., "Safety-belt injuries in children with lap-belt ecchymosis: CT findings in 61 patients," *American Journal of Roentgenography*, 157, (1991), pp. 111–114.

Chest, Abdominal, and Extremity Injuries

OBJECTIVES

When you have completed this chapter you should be able to

▶ Describe the unique characteristics of the child's anatomy as it relates to chest injuries.
▶ Describe the assessment and management of life-threatening chest injuries in children.
▶ List the two abdominal organs most commonly injured in children.
▶ List and describe the most common fractures in children.

Chest Injuries

Chest injury is second to head injury as the leading cause of death from accidental injury in the United States. Thoracic trauma in children is usually blunt, with a wide range of mechanisms of injury that include motor vehicle crashes, either as a pedestrian or as an unrestrained passenger, and bicycle crashes, again as a pedestrian struck or from a handlebar injury to the chest wall. Falls from heights also produce chest injuries. Penetrating injury to the chest comes from plate glass, stones, guns, and knives.

Several unique characteristics of the child's anatomy contribute to the characteristics of chest injuries. The bones and cartilage of the chest are extremely flexible and resilient, accounting for the low incidence of rib fractures in children. However, lung contusions can occur without any evidence of injury to the chest wall. The presence of a rib fracture in a child indicates that there has been a great transfer of energy to underlying lung tissue. A lung contusion and severe injury should be suspected. Children sustain injuries to the bronchi and ruptures of the diaphragm due to blunt crushing forces more frequently than adults.

The organs in the infant's and child's mediastinum (heart, lungs, large blood vessels) are capable of greater movement than found in adults. Wide shifts of these organs can occur with injury that results in dislocation of the heart, compression of the lung, and angulation of the great vessels and of the trachea.

The upper airway is much smaller and prone to obstruction from blood and mucus. Children who sustain major injury swallow air. Gastric distention results and interferes with the diaphragm's movement, further compromising the child's already limited lung volume. Children under 9 years of age are abdominal breathers. If the abdomen fails to move with respiration, a serious abdominal problem may exist.

Assessment and management of chest injuries are part of the initial assessment. Several chest injuries are life-threatening and prompt recognition and response can affect outcome.

Pneumothorax/Hemothorax

Pneumothorax is spontaneous collapse of the lung from blunt or penetrating trauma. It is the most common life-threatening chest injury in children. *Hemothorax* is the accumulation of blood in the pleural space caused by a tear in a blood vessel or lacerated lung. The accumulation of blood in the pleural space causes the lung to collapse. The key symptoms are decreased breath sounds on the side of the injury and respiratory distress. Tachycardia and labored respirations are early signs of respiratory compromise. Cyanosis is a late finding. If hypoperfusion (shock) is present without an apparent bleeding site, consider the possibility of a hemothorax (Figure 11.1).

Tension Pneumothorax

Tension pneumothorax is the progressive entry of air from the lung or through the chest wall into the pleural space that results in lung collapse. It may result from an open chest wound or blunt trauma in which the trachea or bronchi are torn. This produces a shift of the trachea, heart, and esophagus toward the unaffected lung, resulting in angulation of the

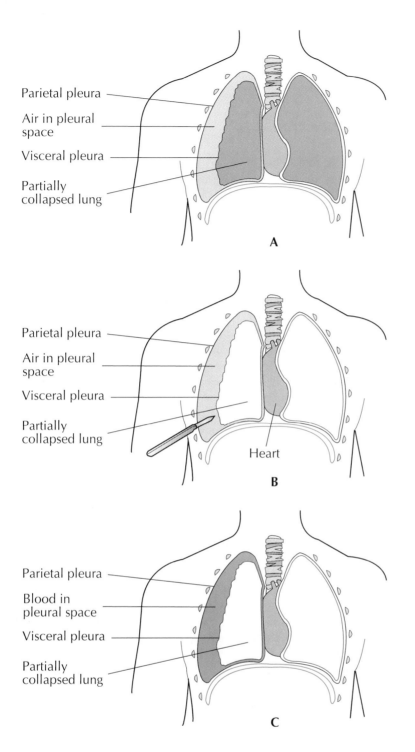

Parietal pleura

Air in pleural space

Visceral pleura

Partially collapsed lung

A

Parietal pleura

Air in pleural space

Visceral pleura

Partially collapsed lung

Heart

B

Parietal pleura

Blood in pleural space

Visceral pleura

Partially collapsed lung

C

FIGURE 11.1   Injuries to the chest: (A) closed pneumothorax, (B) pneumothorax from a penetrating injury, (C) hemothorax.

major blood vessels of the heart and decreased cardiac output. Signs of a tension pneumothorax are decreased breath sounds, paradoxical chest motion, severe dyspnea, subcutaneous emphysema, and hypoperfusion (shock). This is a *true medical emergency.* A child with these signs should be transported immediately to the hospital. Administer high-flow, high-concentration oxygen and cover any open chest wound, taping only 3 corners of the dressing. This injury can be made worse by positive pressure ventilation, ALS management is needle thoracostomy (Figure 11.2).

FIGURE 11.2   Tension pneumothorax.

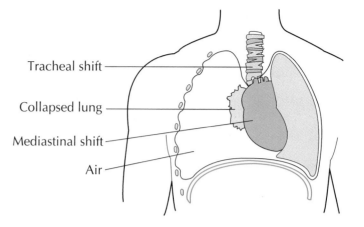

Tracheal shift

Collapsed lung

Mediastinal shift

Air

Cardiac Tamponade

Trauma to the heart and major blood vessels in the chest is uncommon in children. It does occur with penetrating injuries, however. This injury causes bleeding into the pericardial space around the heart, resulting in impairment of the efficient pumping of the heart. Symptoms are distended neck veins, weak pulse, muffled heart sounds, and narrowing pulse pressure. Narrow pulse pressure is the difference between systolic and diastolic pressure observed at a specified interval, for example 90/75 mm Hg. A pulse pressure below 15 mm Hg is critical, indicating an immediate life-threatening emergency. Cardiac arrest is the end result if these symptoms go untreated. This situation requires immediate transport. Treatment is performed at the hospital by inserting a needle into the pericardial space to aspirate the accumulated blood.

Flail Chest

Flail chest, a very rare injury in children, results from multiple rib fractures in sequence, where three or more ribs are each broken in at least two places, creating an unstable chest wall, or the detachment of the sternum. This results in a shifting back-and-forth movement of the major structures—lung, trachea, heart—with every respiration (Figure 11.3). Symptoms are palpable rib fracture, dyspnea, and the flail segment being unstable, thus it moves independently of the chest wall (paradoxical movement). Hospital treatment is required with ventilatory support. Contusion to underlying lung tissue is also a consideration in maintaining effective ventilation.

FIGURE 11.3   *Flail chest.*

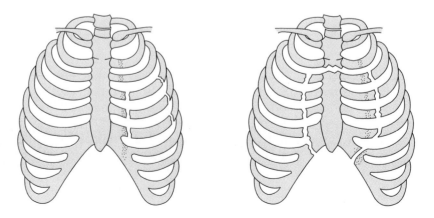

Abdominal Injury

Blunt trauma is the most common cause of injury, and the spleen and liver are the organs most often affected. These injuries result from motor vehicle crashes, falls, child abuse, play, or sports-related injuries. Penetrating injuries are from guns, knives, or impalement on sharp objects.

The unique features of the child's abdominal cavity are that the abdominal organs are slightly large in relation to the abdominal cavity; the undeveloped abdominal muscles offer little protection to a compression or disrupting injury to the liver, spleen, and other organs; and these organs are more exposed to direct trauma because of the broad costal arch (Figure 3.1).

The main concern with abdominal injuries for the prehospital provider is that major abdominal trauma may result in internal hemorrhage and life-threatening hypoperfusion (shock). After the initial assessment is completed, the abdominal assessment, part of the detailed physical exam, is performed keeping the following in mind: Observe the abdomen anteriorly, laterally, and posteriorly for any lacerations, contusions, and distention; gently palpate for pain, rebound tenderness, and guarding.

Spleen

This is the most commonly injured organ in children. Injury to the spleen most often occurs after blunt trauma from a motor vehicle crash, fall, or blow to the flank or torso. Abrasions, ecchymosis, and tenderness suggest the possibility of this injury.

Liver

Injury to the liver occurs almost as frequently as spleen injury. A common mechanism of injury is a blow to the right upper quadrant or chest. Severe hemorrhage can result from vascular injuries inside the liver or injuries to the vena cava and hepatic veins. Symptoms include right upper quadrant pain that may be referred to the shoulder. Rupture of the liver has a high mortality rate with the child presenting in hypoperfusion (shock) and with a tense, distended abdomen.

Pelvis and Perineal Areas

Pelvic trauma usually occurs after trauma from a fall or a motor vehicle crash. Be aware that there can be severe blood loss with a pelvic fracture. Assess femoral pulses. (Note swelling or hematomas.) Palpate pelvic girdle for tenderness or deformity. Inspect genitalia and perineal areas for hematoma. (Blood at the urethra and ecchymosis of the perineum may indicate bladder rupture or pelvic fracture.)

Extremity Injuries

Children are very active and grow at a rapid rate. At times their coordination cannot keep up with the physical demands placed on their bodies; cuts, bruises, and fractures are the result. The types of fractures in children are

AGE GROUP	MECHANISM OF INJURY	TYPES OF INJURY
Infant (6–12 months)		
Rolls over	MVC*: passenger	Brain injury
Creeps, Crawls	Falls: high chair, crib, tables, stairs	Fractures: skull, extremity
Toddler (1–3 years)		
Walking	MVC: passenger, pedestrian	Brain injury
Climbing	Falls: stairs, tables, playgrounds, windows	Fractures: skull, extremity
	Held up, pulled, or lifted up by one arm	Soft-tissue injuries
		Nursemaid's elbow
Preschooler (3–6 years)		
Growth spurts	MVC: pedestrian, passenger bike	Brain injury
Very active	and big wheel	Fractures: skull, pelvis, extremity
Very curious	Falls: playground, windows	
	Lawnmower	
School Age (6–12 years)		
Growth spurts	MVC: pedestrian, passenger bike	Brain injury
Peer pressure	Falls: bike, skateboard, rollerblades	C-spine injury
Accepts dares	Sports	Fractures: skull, pelvis, extremity
		Subluxation of lumbar spine
		Lumbar 1–2, dislocation
		Soft-tissue injuries

*MVC, motor vehicle crash

determined by the child's age, developmental skills, and the season of the year (Table 11.1).

Fractures are not life-threatening, except for amputation or major arterial hemorrhage from a bone fragment severing the vessel. However, skeletal fractures have the potential for producing permanent disability, especially when there is associated nerve and blood vessel damage. When approaching a child with multiple injuries including fractures, the primary survey priorities of airway, breathing, circulatory assessment, neurologic exam, and keeping exposure to a minimum always remain.

Children's bones are unique compared to the adult: they are more porous and more flexible, resulting in different patterns of injury. This results in bone that bends and splinters during the stress of an injury, increasing the risk for soft-tissue damage, as well as vascular and nerve damage. Bone healing occurs faster in children; the younger the child is, the faster the healing process.

Long bones of children grow from a narrow strip of preosseous material called the *epiphyseal plate* at the ends of the bone. Significant injuries to this area of bone result in growth deformities and irregularities of bone length and joint deformities.

Types of Fractures

■ *Bend* fracture: A child's flexible bone can be bent 45° or more before breaking. The bone will straighten slowly, but not completely, to produce some deformity but without the angulation seen when the bone breaks.

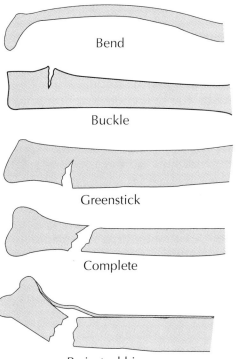

FIGURE 11.4
Types of fractures in children.

Bend

Buckle

Greenstick

Complete

Periosteal hinge

- *Buckle* fracture: This appears as a raised or bulging projection at the fracture site.
- A greenstick fracture is an incomplete fracture similar to the break observed when a green stick is bent and partially breaks.
- A *complete* fracture is one that divides the bone fragments. They often remain attached by a periosteal hinge (Figure 11.4).
- *Epiphyseal* fractures are classified as Salter I through Salter V, with the type of growth disruption increasing from type I through type V (Figure 11.5).

Assessment

- Visually inspect for open wounds, swelling, deformity, and discoloration.
- Feel for the presence of distal pulses.
- Evaluate for pain and the presence of sensation if age appropriate.

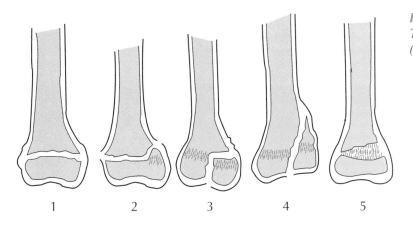

FIGURE 11.5
Types of epiphyseal fractures (Salter classification).

1   2   3   4   5

Open Fracture

Children's bones splinter and may cause pinpoint open wounds (Figure 11.6). Treat any open wound over a fracture as an open fracture. Do not reduce an open fracture, but notify the receiving hospital of the fracture. Treatment of potential infection in the bone must be initiated quickly.

Management of open wounds requires the reduction of contamination and control of bleeding. Flush generously with Ringer's Lactate or Normal Saline. Cover with a sterile gauze roll bandage. Open bleeding wounds require a pressure dressing. Because of the possibility of causing a tourniquet effect resulting in compartment syndrome, do not use elastic bandages for additional pressure.

Potential for Disability

Even though a skeletal injury is not life-threatening, there is the potential for great disability if evaluation of the extremities does not include a neurovascular assessment. (See Chapter 9, "Pediatric Trauma Assessment.")

Splinting Management

Splinting an extremity fracture lessens the possibility of further damage to the nerve, blood vessel, muscle, and skin that may occur with movement of the extremity. Perform the following steps:

- Remove the clothing from around the fracture site.
- Check pulse, capillary refill, skin color and temperature, and sensation in the extremity before and after application of the splint.
- Apply sterile dressings to any open wounds before splinting.
- Immobilize the fracture site above and below the fracture site.
- Splint in the position found; do not try to correct the deformity.
- Take caution with the application of pneumatic splints. They should be clear, if possible, to detect external bleeding. Assess the lower extremities carefully to detect any fracture of the long bones, deformity, instability, ecchymosis, or weak or absent pulses. Any extended length of time in pneumatic splinting may result in vascular compromise, producing compartment syndrome.
- Apply a cold pack.
- Elevate the extremity.

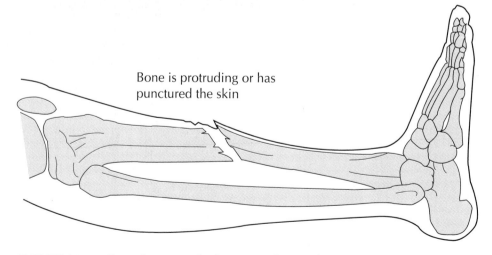

Bone is protruding or has punctured the skin

FIGURE 11.6   Open fracture—the bone may have splintered, protruding through the skin and then withdrawing.

Compartment Syndrome

Compartment syndrome is a true emergency in a child. It is a condition in which the pressure in the closed space of the muscle increases to the point where the blood supply to the muscle fibers is occluded. The pressure is usually caused by hemorrhage, swelling of tissues, or a tight tourniquet-like dressing. It is extremely painful and requires emergency surgical intervention at the hospital.

The primary symptom of compartment syndrome is severe pain. If your assessment does not reveal major extremity injury, perform a neurovascular assessment. Look for changes, such as diminished pulses, poor capillary refill, and decreased sensation in the affected extremity, to alert you to the possibility of compartment syndrome.

Chest, Abdominal, and Extremity Injuries References

Agran, P.F., Castillo, D.N., and Winn, D.G., "Comparison of motor vehicle occupant injuries in restrained and unrestrained 4–14 year olds," *Accident Analysis and Prevention,* 24 (1992), p. 349.

Alexander, M.H., "Mechanism and pattern of injury associated with use of seat belts," *Journal of Emergency Nursing,* 14, no. 4 (August 1988), pp. 214–216.

Allshouse, M.J., and Eichelberger, M.R., "Patterns of Thoracic Injury." In Eichelberger, M.R., ed., *Pediatric Trauma: Prevention, Acute Care, Rehabilitation.* St. Louis: Mosby Year Book, Inc., 1993, pp. 437–448.

Beaver, B.L., Coloibani, P.M., Buck, J.R., et al., "Efficacy of emergency room thoracotomy in pediatric trauma," *Journal of Pediatric Surgery,* 2, (1987), pp. 19–23.

Beaver, B.L., and Laschinger, J.C., "Pediatric thoracic trauma," *Seminars in Thoracic and Cardiovascular Surgery,* 4, no. 3 (July 1992), pp. 255–262.

Corey, E.C., "Blunt and penetrating chest trauma," *Emergency,* 26, no. 4 (April 1994), pp. 34–39.

Glassman, E.S., Johnson, J.R., and Holt, R.T., "Seatbelt injuries in children," *Journal of Trauma,* 33 (1992), p. 822.

Murphy, P.M., and McCammon, L., "Chest trauma," *JEMS,* 18, no. 9 (September 1993), pp. 33–45.

Robertson, W.J., "Crush injury and compartment syndrome." In Eichelberger, M.R., ed., *Pediatric Trauma: Prevention, Acute Care, Rehabilitation.* St. Louis: Mosby Year Book, Inc., 1993, pp. 548–551.

Sivit, C.J., et al., "Safety-belt injuries in children with lap-belt ecchymosis: CT findings in 61 patients," *American Journal of Roentgenography,* 157, (1991), pp. 111–114.

Thomas, M.D., "Musculoskeletal injury." In Eichelberger, M.R., ed., *Pediatric Trauma: Prevention, Acute Care, Rehabilitation.* St. Louis: Mosby Year Book, Inc., 1993, pp. 533–547.

Thompson, W.R., "Patterns of abdominal injury." In Eichelberger, M.R., ed., *Pediatric Trauma: Prevention, Acute Care, Rehabilitation.* St. Louis: Mosby Year Book, Inc., 1993, pp. 451–455.

Burns

OBJECTIVES

When you have completed this chapter you should be able to

▶ Describe common mechanisms of burn injury to children of each developmental age.
▶ Describe the application of the "rule of nines" to children of different ages or sizes.
▶ List the signs indicating the possibility of airway burns.
▶ Identify the burned child needing care in a burn center.
▶ Describe the field management for each of the following types of burns:
  • Thermal
  • Inhalation
  • Chemical
  • Electrical

Epidemiology of Burn Injuries

Burns, the second leading cause of death in children, claim the lives of approximately 1100 children annually in the United States, accounting for approximately 15% of all injury deaths. Burns also leave thousands of children hospitalized, many of whom suffer significantly from the physical and psychological scars of being a burn victim. The average age of burned children is 32 months. Child abuse is suspected in approximately 16% of these cases.

Types of Burns

Thermal Burns

Thermal burns are the result of direct contact with a hot object, flame, or with hot liquids such as water, tea, coffee, or grease.

Scald burns are the most common type of burns in children (Table 12.1). Toddlers like to explore and can easily pull a cup of hot liquid onto their face, neck, arms, and chest. Fortunately, liquids cool quickly and run off, minimizing contact time. Hot grease and thick soup stay in contact with the skin longer, transmitting more heat and resulting in a full-thickness, or third-degree, burn (Figure 12.1).

Immersion into hot water will result in a full-thickness burn after short exposure, depending upon the temperature of the water. The range of exposure time is as follows:

- *2 seconds* when the water temperature is 150°F or higher, hardly enough time to respond and withdraw the extremity, and
- 10 minutes at 120°F in the adult and even less time in the child.

Both the Federal Consumer Product Safety Commission and the plumbing industry have proposed voluntary standards requiring installation of a device that would limit new bathtub and shower hot water heaters to 120°F (50°C), unlikely to cause third-degree burns, except in neonates. Many newly installed hot water heaters have the temperature preset at 120°F.

TABLE 12.1 ■ *Distribution of Children by Age and Burn Type Requiring Treatment in a Burn Center Between 1991 and 1993*

Burn Type	0–2 Years	2–5 Years	5–20 Years
Scald	418 (69.7%)	408 (62.5%)	255 (26.8%)
Flame	45 (7.5%)	133 (20.4%)	578 (60.7%)
Contact	116 (19.3%)	91 (13.9%)	51 (5.3%)
Electrical	4 (0.7%)	11 (1.7%)	43 (4.5%)
All Other Types	17 (2.8%)	10 (1.5%)	26 (2.7%)

Source: Adapted from Saffle, J.R., Davis, B., Williams, P., and the American Burn Association Registry Participant Group, (May/June 1995): "Recent outcomes in the treatment of burn injury in the United States: A report from the American Burn Patient Registry," *Journal of Burn Care Rehabilitation,* 16, no. 3, pp. 219–232.

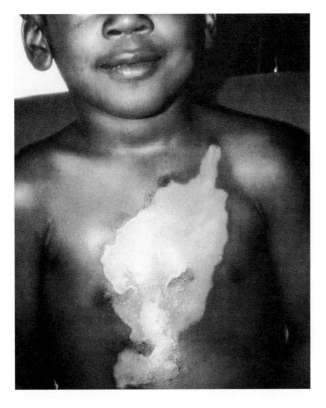

FIGURE 12.1 Arrowhead appearance of a scald burn caused by spilling hot liquid. Note the decreasing width of burn injury as the liquid drained down the chest to form an arrow point.

Flame burns follow scald burns in frequency but are often deadlier. Residential fires are the second highest cause of injury death among children between 1 to 9 years of age. Playing with ignition sources, such as matches, results in the leading cause of fire deaths in children under 5 years of age. The most common cause of early death (within the first hour) from flame burns is respiratory failure due to smoke inhalation.

Fireworks injuries are seasonal and may cause full-thickness burns. Fireworks commonly cause injuries to three body areas:

- The hand, when the firecracker explodes while being held;
- The foot, when the firecracker is dropped; and
- The trunk, when the firecracker explodes in the pocket.

Contact burns can result from direct skin contact with a hot object such as an oven, wood stove, barbecue grill, hot pot or skillet, curling iron or electric rollers, hot pipes, or lighted cigarette. They cause variable tissue damage, depending upon the temperature of the object and contact time. A partial-thickness to full-thickness burn can result, sometimes in the characteristic shape of the object causing the burn. These types of burns can be unintentional or intentional injuries.

Chemical Burns

Chemical burns can result from contact with a variety of solids, liquids, powders, or gases that irritate or burn the skin surface, mucous membranes, or internal organs. They cause variable tissue damage. Lye is especially damaging to the skin, leaving a full-thickness burn as it runs along the skin. Chemical burns also result from ingesting harmful agents such as household products or caustic chemicals. (See Chapter 8, "Poisoning Emergencies," for more information.)

Electrical Burns

Electrical burns result from contact with low-voltage electrical cords or high-voltage tension wires. There are about 1300 fatalities annually in the United States from electrical injury, with pediatric patients accounting for about a third of the victims.

Toddlers can be injured while playing with electrical appliances, sucking on an electrical cord, or, more frequently, playing with wall sockets. There have also been a significant number of incidents involving the use of blow dryers and curling irons, especially in association with bathtub electrocutions. Older children can sustain electrical injuries when struck by lightning or when playing on high-voltage structures.

The degree of tissue damage in electrical burns is related to the number of amps, the length of exposure to the voltage, and the resistance of the tissues. A high-voltage injury can be compared to a crush injury. In addition, the child may be thrown when coming into contact with the electrical current. The injury occurs to large areas of the body and body organs as the current passes through. The heart and central nervous system are especially vulnerable to injury, with a lethal ventricular dysrhythmia resulting if the current crosses the heart at a critical time. Respiratory distress is common, and hypoperfusion (shock) can result from internal bleeding. Moist skin in the antecubital, axillary, and popliteal spaces has a far lower resistance to electrical current, sometimes enough to ignite clothing and result in thermal burns.

Electrical injuries leave an entrance and exit wound. The entrance wound often appears dry, charred, and depressed in the center. Exit wounds often have a "blown-out" appearance. In toddlers, oral burns from chewing on electrical cords have a blown-out appearance. These burns may be significantly deeper, with more tissue destruction than their initial appearance would indicate, and require hospitalization. The eschar (dead tissue) begins to separate between 10 to 14 days, and hemorrhage can occur owing to sloughing of an artery near the wound (Figure 12.2).

Care for the Burn Injury

History

On arrival at the scene, it is important to collect the following information about the child and mechanism of injury:

S   Is the child having any difficulty breathing? What parts of the body are burned? What color is the burned skin? Are there blisters? Has there been any change in the child's mental status? Is the child in pain?

A   Does the child have any known allergies?

M   Does the child regularly take any medications?

P   Does the child have any chronic diseases or serious health problems? If so, what kind? What is the child's approximate weight?

L   When was the child's last oral intake? What was it?

E   How long ago did the burn occur? What caused the burn? (Consider if the mechanism of the burn is suspicious of child abuse.) Was the child enclosed in a closed space with intense heat or smoke? Did the child have any other injury in addition to the burn (e.g., fall, struck by falling objects, etc.)? What treatment has been initiated?

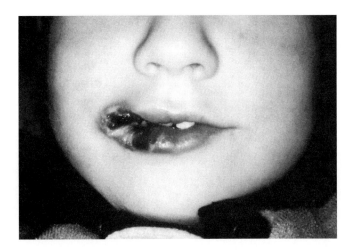

FIGURE 12.2   Burn from biting electrical cord.

Assessment

Depth of Injury

The depth of burns are generally classified as *superficial, partial-thickness,* and *full-thickness.* Another form of classification consists of first-, second-, and third-degree burns (Figure 12.3 and Table 12.2).

A *superficial,* or first-degree, burn affects the epidermis of the skin. It is red, very painful, and blanches readily with pressure. These burns result from a brief contact with a hot liquid or object, flame, or prolonged exposure to sunlight.

A *partial-thickness,* or second-degree, burn affects the epidermis and dermis; however, the hair follicles, sebaceous glands, and sweat glands are not injured. The burn is mottled white to red, moist, and painful with blisters. These burns result from an intense contact with a hot liquid or object, flame, or prolonged overexposure to sunlight.

A *full-thickness, or* third-degree, burn damages the epidermis, dermis, the hair follicles, the sebaceous glands, and sweat glands. Subcutaneous tissues, muscles, bone, and organs may be affected. These burns are commonly painless, white or charred, and leathery in appearance. They result from contact with live steam, chemicals, and prolonged contact with flame or electric current.

Determination of Burn Surface Area

In adults, the "rule of nines" is used to determine the body surface area (BSA) involved. In children, body proportions and body surface area vary by age. The modified rule of nines for children and infants offers a method to calculate burn percentage (Figure 12.4).

An alternate method to assess BSA is to use the child's palm, or clenched fist, which equals 1% of the BSA. The child's palm serves as a guide for quick estimation of the body surface area burned. Remember to use the child's hand and not your own for the BSA calculation.

Assessment of Physiologic Status

Perform the initial assessment and detailed physical exam, looking for signs of an airway injury and other major trauma (Table 12.3). Blunt trauma to the chest may have occurred from a fall or an explosion, resulting in a spontaneous pneumothorax or myocardial contusion.

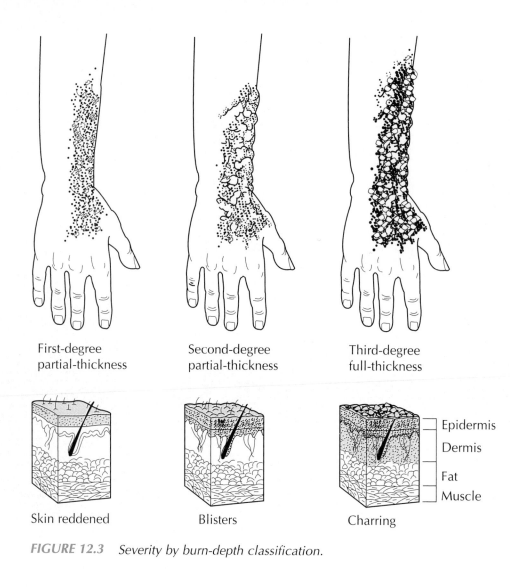

First-degree
partial-thickness

Second-degree
partial-thickness

Third-degree
full-thickness

Epidermis

Dermis

Fat

Muscle

Skin reddened

Blisters

Charring

FIGURE 12.3 *Severity by burn-depth classification.*

TABLE 12.2 ■ *Classification of Burn Severity in Children*

Major Burns
Partial-thickness—20% body surface area (BSA)
Full-thickness > 10% BSA
Burns to hands, face, eyes, ears, feet, genitalia
Airway burn or smoke inhalation suspected
Electrical burns
Additional injuries, signs of hypoperfusion (shock)
Children with chronic health conditions

Moderate Burns
Partial-thickness—10 to 20% BSA
Full-thickness—3 to 10% BSA

Minor Burns
Partial-thickness < 2% BSA
Full-thickness < 2% BSA

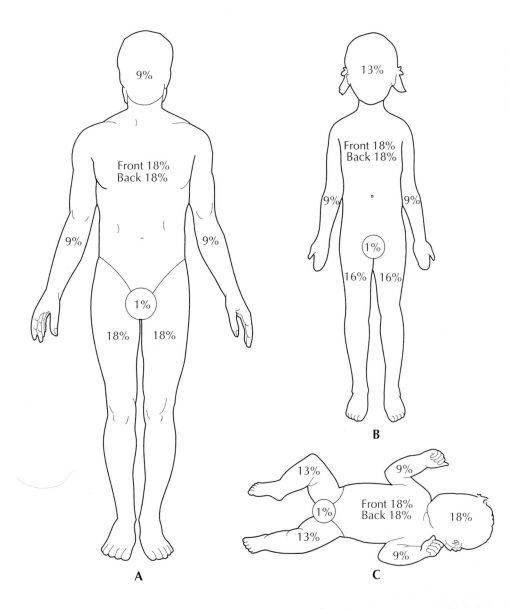

Assess the extent of burn injury and note any circumferential burns, those completely circling the chest or an extremity. Full-thickness circumferential burns around the chest or abdomen may interfere with the child's ability to ventilate.

Signs of hypoperfusion (shock) occurring within 30 minutes of injury suggest an internal hemorrhage from an injury other than the burn. Decreased responsiveness may result from a head injury or hypoxia from smoke inhalation (Figure 12.5).

TABLE 12.3 ■ *Signs and Symptoms of Inhalation Injury*

Child found alert or nonresponsive in a smoke-filled environment.
Singed nasal hair.
Soot in septum, or around the nose and mouth.
Brassy cough, persistent cough.
Sore throat, stridor.
Agitation.
Respiratory distress—cyanosis.

Care for the Burn Injury

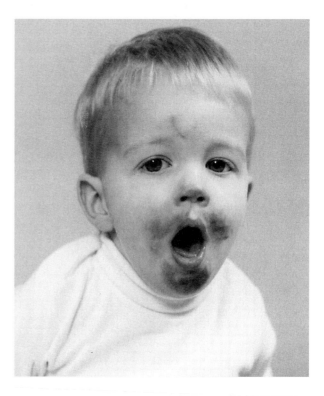

FIGURE 12.5 Suspect an inhalation injury in a child with soot around the nose and mouth and carbonaceous sputum, regardless of level of responsiveness. The child's status could change rapidly.

CAUTION!

Airway Injury

Any child found in an enclosed space or a heavy smoke-filled environment is considered to have an inhalation injury. Exposure to the hot air and toxic fumes, including carbon monoxide, will cause the child's airway to swell and occlude up to 50% of the total airway. Because the swelling process is continuous and rapid, the decision to intubate needs to be determined early, especially if there is a long transport time. BLS providers should rapidly transport this child for airway management or consider ALS intervention.

Management of Thermal Burns

BLS care should include the following:

- Do scene size-up and remove the child from the source of burn injury. *Stop the burning process.* Remove smoldering clothing over and around the burn, but *DO NOT* remove clothing stuck to the burn. Remove jewelry, belt buckles, rings, boots, etc., which may retain heat or hide burns.
- Assess and monitor ABCDEs, especially the airway.
- Administer high-flow, high-concentration oxygen, humidified if possible, by mask, especially if there is a suspicion of inhalation injury. Be prepared to assist ventilations with a bag-valve mask and to administer CPR.
- Keep the child warm. Cover the child's body with a sterile or clean sheet. Burned children are particularly susceptible to hypothermia. When the skin is damaged, it loses its ability to retain heat.

- *DO NOT* use any type of ointment, lotion, or antiseptic on the burned skin.
- For partial-thickness burns, apply cool, wet compresses to small areas for pain control if within 2 hours of injury. Cover no more than 15% of the body surface area at any time with cool, wet compresses to reduce the chance of hypothermia.
- For full-thickness burns, *DO NOT* wash or apply cool, wet compresses. Cover the burned area with a dry sterile sheet.
- *DO NOT* apply ice or rupture blisters. Ice may cause further tissue damage.
- Elevate the head 30° to assist breathing if no head injury is suspected. Elevate the burned extremity.
- Rapidly transport the child to the appropriate hospital so the child can get to a burn center, if available, in cases of major injury. *DO NOT* delay, especially with inhalation injury (Table 12.4).

ALS providers may initiate the following additional care:

- If performing endotracheal intubation, choose an endotracheal tube two sizes smaller than what would usually be used for this child. Remember that the mucous membranes of the airway are swollen and highly vulnerable to injury from intubation.
- If the burn covers more than 15% BSA, or there is other trauma, start an IV of Ringer's Lactate or Normal Saline at a rate of 10 ml/kg/per hour or as specified in local protocols. Use an extremity without burns for the IV, if available, to avoid contamination of the wound.
- If signs of hypoperfusion (shock) are present, give Ringer's Lactate or Normal Saline, 20 ml/kg IV push. If vital signs do not improve after 5 minutes, repeat the bolus of Ringer's Lactate or Normal Saline. Up to three boluses may be needed in severe shock.

Management of Chemical Burns

All prehospital providers should administer the following care for *chemical burns to the skin:*

- Protect yourself by using protective devices and clothing specified by OSHA standards.
- For water-soluble chemicals, place the child in the shower or otherwise flush the burned surface with copious amounts of water. Remove the child's clothing while in the shower, taking care to brush off powder and solid chunks prior to the flushing. Continue flushing until all the chemical has been removed.

TABLE 12.4 ■ *Characteristics of Burns that Should Be Evaluated at the Hospital*

Burns greater than 10% body surface area (BSA).
Burns that involve the face, hands, feet, or genitalia even if the burn is less than 10% BSA.
All electrical and chemical burns, especially if the chemical was ingested.
Burns with smoke-inhalation injury.
Burns associated with other injury.

- For chemicals that are not water soluble, take the following alternate actions:

Chemical and Its Characteristics	Management
Phenol—poorly soluble in water	Remove clothing, flush with water, then apply baby oil or other oily substance.
Sodium metal—reacts with water by burning	Brush off and apply petroleum jelly to affected skin.
Sulfuric acid—higher concentrations cause greater damage	Use soap and water, rinse with copious amounts of water.

- Cover burns with a clean sheet and keep the child warm.
- Transport patient rapidly to the hospital.

All emergency personnel should provide the following care for *chemical burns to the eyes:*

- Immediately flush with large amounts of saline or water for 20 minutes.
- Cover injured eye with a patch.
- Transport rapidly.

Refer to Chapter 8, "Poisoning Emergencies," for management of chemical ingestions.

Management of Electrical Burns

BLS field care for *low-voltage electrical burns* includes the following:

- Protect yourself. Attempt to disconnect the power source and remove the child from contact.
- Assess and monitor ABCDEs.
- Administer high-flow, high-concentration oxygen.
- Place a clean dressing over entrance and exit burn sites.
- Assess and manage other injuries.
- Transport patient to hospital.

BLS field care for *high-voltage electrical burns* includes:

- Protect your own safety. Attempts to remove high-voltage electrical wires from the child by using ropes or wooden poles can be very dangerous. Notify the power company immediately to turn off the power prior to extrication. If the child is thrown clear, remove child to an area of greater safety.
- Perform the initial assessment and monitor ABCs.
- Stabilize the cervical spine and maintain the airway.
- Ventilate with high-flow, high-concentration oxygen.
- Perform CPR if indicated. Consider the need for automated external defibrillation.
- Perform detailed physical exam.
- Cover burn sites with sterile dressing. Look for entrance and exit wounds.
- Keep the child warm.
- Immediately transport to hospital. Injuries are often more severe than external signs indicate.

ALS personnel should additionally provide the following care, according to local protocols:

- Intubate the child if airway control is inadequate.
- Attach a pulse oximeter and a cardiac monitor. Record a rhythm strip.
- Initiate defibrillation if the child is in ventricular fibrillation or asystole.
- Start an IV of Ringer's Lactate or Normal Saline at a keep-open rate.

Child Abuse and Burn Injury

Children under 5 years of age represent the age group most often found with burns resulting from child abuse. There are characteristic burns that should make you suspicious of the possibility of child abuse. The child presenting with burns to the back, buttocks, and posterior neck should alert your suspicion of abuse. The child who unintentionally knocks over a cup of hot liquid onto himself has an arrowhead-shaped spill pattern over the anterior shoulder, chest, and possibly the face.

Circumferential scald burns of hands or feet that are clearly demarcated and uniform with no splash marks are telltale signs of abuse. When the hands or feet are held forcibly under hot running water, there are characteristic burns to the backs of hands or top of the feet. Burns limited to the genitalia and buttocks, with skin folds unburned, occur when children are dipped and held in a tub of hot water. This commonly occurs when parents are frustrated with toilet training. (See Chapter 13, "Child Abuse," for more details.)

Burns References

Ball, J., and Bindler, R., *Pediatric Nursing: Caring for Children.* Norwalk, CT: Appleton & Lange, (1995), pp. 705–716.

Ball, R.A., "Hot stuff: Assessing and treating burns," *JEMS*, 18, no. 2 (February 1993), pp. 30–41.

Bourne, M.K., "Fire and smoke: Managing skin and inhalation burns," *JEMS*, 14, no. 9 (September 1989), pp. 62–82.

Cherington, M., Martorano, F., Siebuhr, L., Stieg, R., and Yarnall, P., "Childhood lightning injuries on the playing field," *JEMS*, 12, no. 1 (January 1994), pp. 39–41.

Clark, J.R., "Managing burns in children," *JEMS*, 15, no. 4 (April 1990), pp. 90–94.

Fontanarosa, P.B., "Taking charge of patients with electrical injuries," *JEMS*, 17, no. 3 (March 1992), pp. 50–70.

Hall, M.L., and Sills, R.M., "Electrical and lightning injuries." In Barkin, R.M., ed., *Pediatric Emergency Medicine: Concepts and Clinical Practice.* St. Louis: Mosby Year Book, Inc., 1992, pp. 418–429.

Herndon, D.N., Rutan, R.L., and Rutan, T.C., "Management of the pediatric patient with burns," *Journal of Burn Care and Rehabilitation,* 14, no. 1 (January/February 1993), pp. 3–8.

Manoguerra, A.S., "Fire toxicology," *Emergency*, 26, no. 7 (July 1994), pp. 20–26.

Mistovich, J.J., and Eley, M., "When lightning strikes," *Emergency*, 23, no. 6 (June 1991), pp. 22–25.

Morbidity and Mortality Weekly Report, "Deaths resulting from residential fires—United States, 1991," *Morbidity and Mortality Weekly Report*, 43, no. 49 (December 16, 1994), pp. 901–904.

Parish, R.A., "Thermal burns." In Barkin, R.M., ed., *Pediatric Emergency Medicine: Concepts and Clinical Practice.* St. Louis: Mosby Year Book, Inc., 1992, pp. 424–429.

Saffle, J.R., Davis, B., Williams, P., and the American Burn Association Registry Participant Group, "Recent outcomes in the treatment of burn injury in the United States: A report from the American Burn Patient Registry," *Journal of Burn Care Rehabilitation,* 16, no. 3, (May/June 1995): pp. 219–232.

Woosnam, J., "Firefighter, save my child!" *Emergency,* 19, no. 6 (June 1995), pp. 46–50.

13

Child Abuse

OBJECTIVES

When you have completed this chapter you should be able to

▶ Distinguish between physical abuse, sexual abuse, emotional abuse, and neglect.
▶ Describe the range of injuries seen in physically and sexually abused children.
▶ Demonstrate the appropriate method for handling a parent or care provider in a suspected abuse situation.
▶ Describe the procedure by state law for reporting suspected child abuse.
▶ Demonstrate appropriate documentation of findings in suspected child-abuse cases.

Definition and Description of the Problem

Child abuse is a complex health and social problem that is on the rise in today's society; it knows no socioeconomic boundaries. The major difference between child abuse and unintentional injury is that in the former the child is injured or allowed to be injured by his or her parent, guardian, or caregiver.

Personal feelings are the greatest obstacle to the successful management of child abuse and neglect. You and your coworkers are often the first individuals in a position to gather information that will later determine whether the hospital care providers are dealing with child abuse or an accidental injury.

> Since repeat abuse occurs in more than 20% of all children, often leading to permanent injury and death, only early recognition of child abuse will allow the interruption of the vicious cycle which may not only kill the involved child but siblings as well. (Kottmeier, 1987, p. 343)

Proper documentation and reporting of your suspicions of neglect and/or abuse may be the only means of assuring that action will be taken to reduce the child's risk. Accusations and confrontation at the scene will delay treatment, and in some cases, the parents or care providers may refuse transport of the child. Objective documentation of the environment and the events is often the only evidence strong enough to justify removal of the child from the household, thus stopping the cycle of abuse.

Epidemiology

- In infants under 6 months of age, child abuse is second only to SIDS as the leading cause of death.
- Up to 20% of all traumatic injuries seen in children 3 years of age or younger are caused by maltreatment; however, a third of all child-abuse cases are reported in children over 3 years of age.
- Between 2000 to 5000 children die each year as a result of child-abuse injuries.

Psychosocial Contributors to Child Abuse

A large number of abused and neglected children suffer permanent physical and emotional disabilities, and a large number of these go unreported yearly.

The abusive situation is often precipitated by a crisis, which might be a minor problem that sets off the abuser. It is usually associated with a long series of frustrations or the abuser's inability to cope with problems, such as poverty, unemployment, or too many children. Additionally, factors that can contribute to the abuse of a child include marital disharmony or social isolation, a single parent who is isolated or lacking social support, and drug and/or alcohol abuse.

In some cases, the child has certain characteristics that place him or her at higher risk for abuse. The child may be singled out for abuse because he or she is viewed as "different"—such as having a chronic illness, premature birth, or a physical deformity. Hyperactive or difficult-to-manage children are also at high risk for abuse. Sometimes the child may simply resemble a relative or ex-spouse disliked by the abuser.

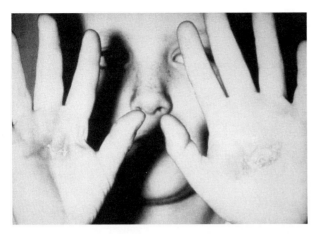

FIGURE 13.1 Small, round burns caused by a cigarette held to the skin.

Classifications of Child Abuse

Physical Abuse

Physical abuse results in trauma to the soft tissue, skeleton, central nervous system, abdominal organs, or teeth. The injuries may be inflicted by beatings, burns, shaking, throwing the child against a wall or on the ground, binding, gagging, twisting extremities, poisoning, or starvation. Overly harsh discipline that results in injury is also considered physical abuse.

Signs of physical abuse include the following characteristic patterns of soft-tissue and skeletal injuries:

- Small round burns or scars, often from cigarettes (Figure 13.1).
- Glove or stocking burns from immersion of the hands or feet in hot water. These burns have a characteristic lack of splash marks (Figure 13.2). (Refer to Chapter 12, "Burns.")
- Burns to buttocks, legs, and feet, often with creases behind the knees and upper thighs spared. These burns occur most commonly

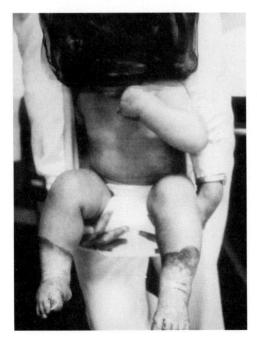

FIGURE 13.2 "Stocking" burns caused by immersion of the feet into hot water. Note the distinct line of the burn on the legs. The lack of splash marks indicates the child was restrained in the hot water and could not escape.

FIGURE 13.3 *Burns to buttocks, legs, and feet with creases behind the knees and in upper thighs spared. This immersion burn often occurs as punishment for soiling underclothes during toilet training.*

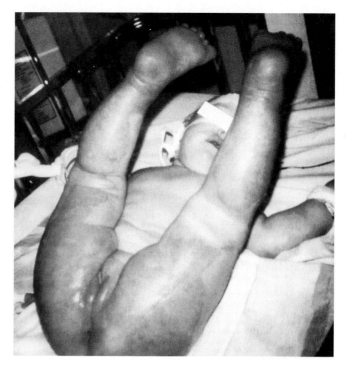

in infants and toddlers who soil themselves during toilet training (Figure 13.3).

■ Demarcated burns in shape of object used, such as an iron, stove burner, oven rack, or radiator (Figure 13.4).

■ Slap marks resembling the shape of a hand.

■ Welts showing shape of tool used—belts, buckles, hangers, electrical cords (loop marks), or chains (Figure 13.5).

■ Suspicious bruises in various stages of healing (Table 3.3). Active children often have bruises over bony prominences (shins, hips, spine, lower arms, forehead, and under the chin) caused by falls and bumping into objects during play. Suspicious sites for bruises are on the upper arms, trunk, upper anterior legs, sides of the face, ears and neck, genitalia, and buttocks (Figure 13.6)

■ Human bite marks indicating the pattern of teeth and size of an adult's mouth. Pay particular attention to the characteristics of teeth marks (chips and space between teeth).

■ Marks indicating the child has been bound or gagged.

FIGURE 13.4 *Demarcated burns in shape of object used, in this case an iron. (From* Atlas of Pediatric Physical Diagnosis *by Davis Zitelli, 1987, Mosby International, London, UK. Reprinted with permission.)*

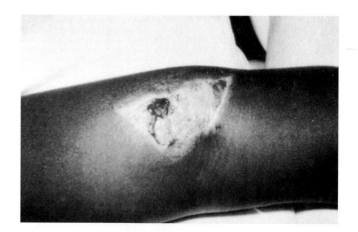

Chapter 13: Child Abuse

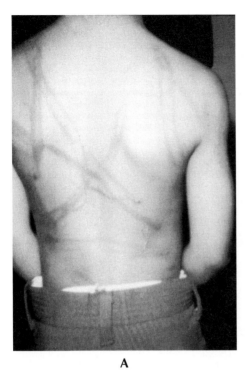

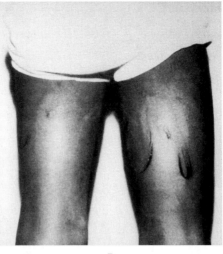

B

FIGURE 13.5   Welt in the shape of the item used for beating. (A) welt caused by a willow branch. (B) Welt caused by a looped electrical cord;

A

- Fractures may be detected by poor alignment or the child's sudden unwillingness to use an extremity. X rays of long bones taken at the hospital may reveal numerous fractures in various stages of healing (Figure 13.7).

Shaken Baby Syndrome

Sometimes caretakers become so frustrated with an infant that they shake the baby, not realizing that this action can cause serious injury. After the shaking, the baby often is thrown down, compounding the injury. The blood vessels in the baby's brain are torn as the brain strikes the skull, resulting in bruising and intracranial bleeding. There may be no physical marks on the infant, but the baby will have signs of increased intracranial pressure such as seizures, respiratory arrest, unequal pupils,

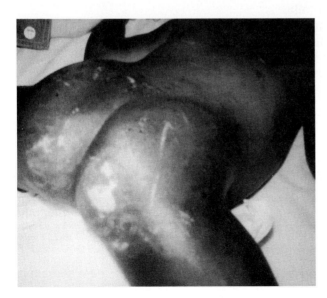

FIGURE 13.6   Bruising on the buttocks from repeated spankings.

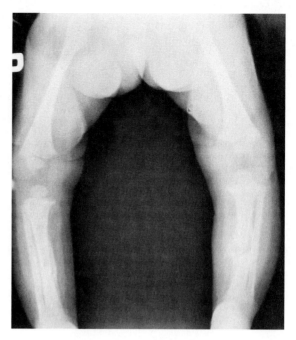

FIGURE 13.7 *X-ray picture of the legs. Note fresh fractures on right tibia and fibula as well as healing fracture on left tibia.*

and/or posturing. If the infant is dead at the scene, you may suspect sudden infant death syndrome (SIDS). However, the mechanism of injury will be determined by autopsy.

Sexual Abuse

Sexual abuse is defined as any sexual contact between a child and another person in a position of authority, no matter the age, where the child's participation was obtained through threats, bribery, coercion, or similar tactics. These sexual contacts can include sexual assault or physical force, but they are not limited only to intercourse. Fondling, sodomy, exhibitionism, pornography, and prostitution are also considered forms of sexual abuse.

Often the signs of sexual abuse in young children are subtle because fondling may not result in apparent injury. Some of the more overt signs of sexual abuse include the following:

- Bruising on the genitalia.
- Lacerations indicating vaginal and/or anal penetration.
- Semen on clothes or body.
- Discharge from the vagina or penis, perhaps associated with a sexually transmitted disease.
- Bruising around the mouth or a tear of the frenum.

Neglect

Neglect involves the willful or unintentional absence of care for a child's basic life necessities, which places the child's life or health in jeopardy. These include lack of adequate nutrition, leading to poor growth and development; lack of medical care; lack of psychosocial support; or lack of education. Abandonment and/or lack of committed and consistent daily care is also considered neglect. Signs of neglect include the following:

- The child is unbathed and wearing unusually dirty clothing or has poor hygiene.

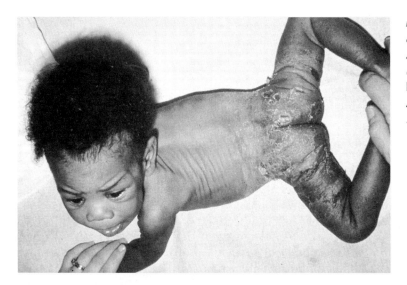

FIGURE 13.8 *The neglected infant often appears poorly nourished, small, and underweight for the reported age. (From Atlas of Pediatric Physical Diagnosis by Davis Zitelli, 1987, Mosby International, London, UK. Reprinted with permission.)*

- The child is poorly nourished, small, and underweight for age (Figure 13.8).
- The child is inappropriately dressed for the season or weather.
- There seems to be an inappropriate delay in seeking medical care.

Emotional Abuse

Emotional abuse is the most difficult of the four classifications to identify and often goes unreported. It involves the failure of caregivers to provide a child with the support necessary for the development of a sound personality. This may occur by intimidation, subtle or overt rejection, threats, or excessive criticism.

Care of the Suspected Child-Abuse Victim

It is vitally important that you remember the following steps when managing a suspected abuse victim:

- Your primary responsibility is to manage the injuries rather than place blame.
- Document history and observations in an *objective* rather than a subjective manner.
- Remain nonjudgmental in the presence of the child's caregivers at all times.

History

In addition to the routine history you would obtain for any child with an injury, some additional questions should be asked. Questions should be phrased to obtain facts about the incident so that no apparent blame can be perceived by the caregiver.

- How did the injury occur? How long ago did it happen?
- Who was with the child or found the child at the time of injury? Did anyone witness the incident?
- Has the child been moved from the site of the injury?

Assessment

Indications of abuse may be severe or deceptively mild, making your assessment difficult. Remember that many clues to child abuse lie in the assessment of the home; inappropriate attitude of the caregiver toward the child's injuries, or of the child's reactions to the injury; and changes in the history or account of the injury given by the caregiver over time.

Parental Behavior

Uneasy, unsure, or uncertain behavior on the part of the family member reporting the history of the injury is sometimes your first clue to a child-abuse case. Though the abusive parent or caregiver usually has requested your assistance, this individual may react with anger, fear, withdrawal, hostility, or silence to questions about the history of the injury. Overreaction to or unusual lack of concern about the injury is sometimes noted as well, but this is difficult to document without seeming subjective. Oftentimes there is a delay in seeking treatment. This delay may be because the severity of the child's injury is just now apparent, or in some cases the abuser has left the scene allowing others to call for help. Pay close attention to the behavior the parent or caregiver shows toward the child. These individuals may become angry, indifferent, fault the child, or provide little, if any, support or consolation.

Child's Behavior

The child may also show unusual behavior such as the following:

- Demonstrating no expectation of being comforted by the parent or caregiver.
- Being overly friendly toward strangers or less afraid of strangers when compared to other children his or her own age;
- Having a withdrawn or diminished response to pain.

There may also be some evidence of developmental delay, overt anger and hostility, mistrust, or sexual acting out. Abused children typically will not betray their parents by describing the abuse.

Environmental Clues

Clues of abuse may be found at the scene, and because you may be the only health care provider to see the child's environment before it is "cleaned up," it is important to document in a factual manner what you observe in the home.

- Are there signs of a struggle or destruction?
- Are family members and/or neighbors discussing who or how the child was injured?
- Is there evidence of drugs or alcohol?
- Is there evidence of the reported accident and does it seem probable for the environment and developmental skills of the child?

Abuse may be suspected if the following items or combination of items are noted:

- A child has noticeable injuries that the parent or care provider doesn't mention.
- The child's injuries and/or age indicates a better explanation than is being offered.

- Your physical findings do not match the history given.
- Information about the injury changes with further questioning.

Scene Size-Up

Observe the details of the child's environment, especially for little clues that may be useful in proving neglect or abuse. Remember, this situation is potentially volatile and dangerous. You may need law enforcement assistance to facilitate patient care. If the scene situation deteriorates to the point where personal injury may result, use good judgment rather than be ruled by your emotions. Retreat to a position of safety.

Providing appropriate medical care is a priority in cases of suspected abuse, *not* proving or disproving that child abuse exists at that moment. The determination of a neglectful or abusive situation is usually made after the incident is over. Data from EMS, law enforcement, hospital personnel, and child protection services are compared and a conclusion is reached in juvenile court.

Management

- Perform scene size-up.
- Conduct initial assessment and check ABCs.
- Treat any major injuries.
- Remove child from situation and transport to hospital.
- Keep the following communication guidelines in mind when at the scene:
  1. *DO NOT* approach the parent or care provider in an accusatory manner.
  2. *DO NOT* judge the parents; someone else may be the perpetrator.
  3. *DO NOT* separate the child from the parents unless the child is in immediate danger. The child is still fearful of separation, even if the parent is the abuser.
- Appropriately document in a factual manner everything heard or observed. See guidelines for documentation below.
- Report suspected abuse to hospital personnel upon arrival at the hospital. *DO NOT* convey sensitive information over the radio. Hospital personnel can set appropriate social services into motion to protect the child and support the family.
- Report suspected abuse to those authorities required by your state's law. You could be sued for negligence if you do not.

Documentation

Record the child's condition and physical injuries as you would for any other case; however, recognize that this record may well wind up in court. As already stated, it is particularly important in cases of suspected child abuse to record your observations in an *objective* manner; subjective reporting is often disregarded. Here are some guidelines:

- Describe injuries by appearance, shape, color, size, location, and stage of healing, rather than stating your impression of the object that caused the injury. For example: A burn that you suspect was caused by a cigarette should be described by its appearance—a circular burn, approximately 1/2 inch in diameter, red and weeping.
- Draw pictures of shapes of injuries (burns, bruises, lacerations, etc.) and their location on the body. These drawings do not have to be of artist's quality to convey information.

- Record statements of all persons at the scene as direct quotations, not your summary of what was said. Include any apparent discrepancies in history among those present.
- Describe the setting in which you found the child, as well as the setting of the incident if the child has been moved. You and your coworkers are likely to be the only health care providers to see the environment before all evidence has been cleaned up. You alone can provide a window to the environment for medical and social services personnel to better recognize the case as true abuse.
- Record both the parents' and child's behavior and their interaction with each other.

Reactions of the EMS Provider

It is common for the prehospital care provider to have strong emotional reactions to child-abuse situations. It can be difficult to contain your feelings of anger, frustration, and disbelief at the horror of the situation, and these feelings may get in the way of your physical assessment, reaction toward the family or care provider, and documentation of the situation.

Remember that you are the child's advocate. If you act or appear judgmental toward the parents, they may not let you take the child to the hospital. Difficult as the situation may be, remember that the only way you can help the child, other than providing care for the injuries, is to remove the child from the scene and transport the child to the hospital and to safety. Remain nonjudgmental, document the facts, and report your suspicions to the receiving hospital personnel.

Once you have delivered the child to the receiving hospital personnel, your feelings may intensify. If so, you need to deal with them for your own emotional well-being. This is an appropriate time to discuss those feelings with personnel at the hospital, such as a physician, nurse, social worker, your partner, or other members of your support group. *Be careful to discuss only your feelings rather than the actual information you have collected about the scene.* Remember that confidentiality is important in the work you do and the patients you manage, regardless of the nature of the call. (See Chapter 17, "Crisis and Stress Management," for suggestions to help with managing such an emotionally charged case.)

Child Abuse References

Berkowitz, C.D., "Pediatric abuse: New patterns of injury," *Emergency Clinics of North America,* 13, no. 2 (May 1995), pp. 321–341.

Brown, G.R., et al., "Diagnosing child maltreatment," *North Carolina Medical Journal,* 55, (September 1994), pp. 404–408.

Butts, J.D., "Injuries, description, documentation, evidence issues," *North Carolina Medical Journal,* 55, (September 1994), pp. 423–427.

Crouse, K.A., "Munchausen syndrome by proxy: Recognizing the victim," *American Journal of Nursing,* 93, no. 6 (June 1992), pp. 249–250.

Devlin, B.K., and Reynolds, E., "Child abuse: How to recognize it, how to intervene," *American Journal of Nursing,* 94, no. 3 (March 1994), pp. 26–31.

Dorfman, D.H., and Paradise, J.E., "Emergency diagnosis and management of physical abuse and neglect of children," *Current Opinion in Pediatrics,* 7, (1995), pp. 297–301.

Levin, A.V., "Child abuse: Challenges and controversies," *Pediatric Emergency Care,* 3, (Fall 1987) pp. 211–217.

Newborn Management

OBJECTIVES

When you have completed this chapter you should be able to

▶ Describe the important parameters for assessment of the newborn.
▶ Describe the four mechanisms of heat loss in a newborn infant and ways to manage each.
▶ List causes of respiratory distress in the newborn.
▶ Describe airway management of the newborn.
▶ Describe appropriate oxygen administration to the newborn.

Physiologic Adaptations at Birth

The fetus exists in an environment of amniotic fluid that is primarily composed of urine and fetal lung fluid until labor and delivery. Newborns must rapidly make a transition to the outside world from a temperature-controlled, protected environment in utero. Newborns must make three major physiologic adaptations necessary for survival:

- Changing their circulatory pattern.
- Emptying fluid from their lungs and beginning ventilation;
- Maintaining body temperature.

Most newborns make this transition with minimal support. Only 6% of full-term newborns need some resuscitation, but the percentage increases for low birth-weight infants.

The newborn's chest is usually compressed during a vaginal delivery, which forces some of the fluid in the lungs out through the mouth and nose. The chest wall recoils after delivery and draws air into the lungs. The initial breath is stimulated by the newborn's response to hypoxia, acidosis, and temperature.

When the umbilical cord is cut, fetal circulation that bypassed the lungs is abruptly ended. As the lungs expand with the initial breaths, resistance to blood flow in the lungs' blood vessels is decreased, making it easier for blood to flow through them. At the same time, the resistance to blood flow in the extremities is increased. This sets the stage for the newborn's blood to be oxygenated by the lungs rather than through the placenta. (See Table 14.1 for causes of hypoxia in newborns.)

Newborns have a large body surface area (BSA) for their weight, decreased tissue insulation, and a poorly developed temperature regulation mechanism. Their head is proportionately larger and accounts for 20% of BSA. In addition, newborns enter the world wet, which promotes rapid heat loss. Delivery into a cool environment only increases the heat loss suffered by the infant. (See Table 14.2 for mechanisms of heat loss in newborns.)

Newborns attempt to conserve heat by maintaining a flexed position and vasoconstriction. Hypothermia develops rapidly in the newborn if not quickly managed. To produce heat, the infants raise their metabolic rate by breaking down fat cells. The stress of heat production places the baby at greater risk for hypoxia, acidosis, bradycardia, and hypoglycemia.

TABLE 14.1 ■ *Causes of Hypoxia in the Newborn*

CONDITIONS DURING LABOR AND DELIVERY	CONDITIONS PRESENT OR DEVELOPING AFTER BIRTH
Compression of the umbilical cord during delivery	Airway obstruction from secretions or meconium
Stress from a difficult labor and delivery	Hypothermia and cold stress
Maternal hemorrhage from placenta previa or placenta abruptio	Large blood loss
	Immature lungs in a premature infant

TABLE 14.2 ■ *Mechanisms of Heat Loss in Newborns and Appropriate Management*

MECHANISMS OF HEAT LOSS	TEMPERATURE CONTROL MANAGEMENT
Evaporation: Heat loss from moisture vaporizing from the skin surface.	Dry the skin surface. Cover with dry towel or blanket. Wrap in cellophane or bubble wrap.
Conduction: Heat loss into a cold surface on which the baby is placed.	Use warm blankets or towels. Place on mother's abdomen and cover. Cover head.
Convection: Heat loss to the cooler air circulating and moving over the infant.	Prevent exposure to air currents. Cover the infant's head. Avoid use of cool oxygen.
Radiation: Heat loss to cooler objects not in direct contact with the infant.	Heat the ambulance interior prior to transport. Place heat packs around the baby, *not in direct contact with the skin.*

Imminent Delivery

When called to care for an obstetrical emergency, you have both the mother and at least one newborn as patients. One person should have primary responsibility to care for the mother while the other prehospital provider cares for the newborn. In this way, neither patient will be forgotten in the excitement of the birth.

If you arrive on the scene prior to delivery, it is necessary to determine if time exists to transport the mother to the nearest hospital. It is of course preferable that the delivery occur at the hospital under controlled circumstances, with all needed equipment and personnel to care for both the mother and infant.

History

To determine how much time you have for transport before delivery may occur, ask the questions in regular type. When you will manage the delivery, or the baby was born prior to your arrival, add the questions in italics to the history.

S   When did labor begin? What are the frequency and length of contractions? How many minutes are there between contractions? Has the mother's water broken? Does she have the urge to move her bowels? Does she feel the need to push? Has there been any vaginal bleeding?

A   *Does the mother have any allergies?*

M   *Did the mother use street drugs during the pregnancy? When was the last dose taken?*

P   Were there complications with prior pregnancies? Did she have a prior C-section? Has she had prenatal care? *Has she seen a doctor regularly for prenatal care?* How many children has she had previously? *Does the mother have any illnesses or need special care for a chronic disease during her pregnancy?*

L   *When was the mother's last oral intake? What was it?*

E   What is the mother's due date? How many weeks pregnant is the mother? *If the infant has already been born, ask the mother or birth attendant how long ago the birth occurred and whether the baby breathed immediately.*

Assessment

Delivery is imminent when the mother's contractions are 2 minutes or less apart, her water has broken, and she has an urge to move her bowels. If crowning is evident after inspecting the mother's perineal area, prepare for delivery prior to transport. Decisions to transport for less imminent delivery should be based upon transport time to the nearest hospital and local protocols. Vaginal bleeding is a sign of early separation of the placenta from the uterus, an emergency that places the mother and newborn in danger. Immediate transport is required.

Management

BLS care for the mother with impending delivery includes the following:

- Use body substance isolation procedures.
- Designate one provider to care for the mother while the other provider cares for the infant.
- Collect all needed supplies to care for the infant, including warm towels if available.
- Heat the ambulance to protect the newborn from hypothermia.
- Follow guidelines for care of the newborn beginning on page 208.
- If the mother is transported to the hospital prior to delivery, place her on her left side. Monitor her ABCs and progress in labor. Administer oxygen by face mask.
- For ALS care and the management of labor and delivery complications, refer to appropriate paramedic textbooks.

Care of the Newly Born Infant

Newborns often need only supportive care to make the transition from fetus to independent life. Those newborns needing more extensive resuscitation are born to mothers with complications such as premature labor, improper presentation of the newborn, hemorrhage, substance abuse, and chronic illnesses such as diabetes.

Assessment

Most full-term newborns present to the world head first, covered with blood and amniotic fluid. The baby appears long and skinny, and the skin is generally dry, flaky, and wrinkled. The baby makes spontaneous movements of the extremities but maintains the arms and legs in a flexed, fetal position. Cyanosis of the hands and feet is common when the newborn is trying to conserve heat. Cyanosis of the mucous membranes indicates hypoxia or a congenital heart defect.

Assessment and management of the newborn are usually performed together. As with any initial assessment, airway is the primary concern, followed by the initiation of breathing and maintenance of the heart rate. Prevention of hypothermia should be done simultaneously with the initial assessment. (See Table 14.3 for normal birth weights and vital signs of the full-term newborn.) The APGAR score is commonly taken at 1 and 5 minutes after birth to evaluate the baby's respiratory, circulatory, and neurologic systems and the need for supportive care. The five categories evaluated include color, pulse, grimace, muscle tone, and respiratory effort. (See Table 14.4 for the APGAR scoring criteria.)

TABLE 14.3 ■ *Normal Vital Signs for Full-term Newborns*

Birth weight (37–40 week gestation)	5–10 lb (2.2–4.5 kg), average is 7.5 lb (3.5 kg)
Heart rate	120–160/min
Respiratory rate	30–60/min
Systolic blood pressure	55–75 mm Hg
Temperature	96.8°F–98.6°F

TABLE 14.4 ■ *APGAR Scoring Criteria*

CHARACTERISTIC EVALUATED	SCORE		
	0	**1**	**2**
Appearance (color)	Blue or pale	Body pink, extremities blue	Completely pink
Pulse rate	Absent	< 100/min	> 100/min
Grimace (reflex irritability)	No response	Grimace	Cough or sneeze
Activity (muscle tone)	Limp	Some flexion of extremities	Active movement
Respiratory effort	Absent	Slow or irregular	Good crying

KEY: *Directions for Administration of the APGAR*

Appearance (color) reflects peripheral tissue oxygenation. For nonwhite newborns, it is important to inspect the color of the mucous membranes of the mouth and conjunctiva, as well as the color of the lips, palms of the hands, and soles of the feet.

Pulse rate should be counted for at least 30 seconds for accuracy.

Grimace (reflex irritability) is judged by the infant's response to passing a catheter into the tip of the nose after suctioning. It can also be evaluated by slapping the sole of the foot with the palm of your hand. The usual response from a healthy newborn is a loud, angry cry.

Activity (muscle tone) refers to the degree of flexion and resistance offered by the infant when you attempt to extend the extremities. Any attempt to alter the normal flexed position of the extremities should be met by resistance.

Respiratory effort evaluates the adequacy of ventilation. Look for slow, shallow, irregular, or gasping respirations, which would be scored as 1.

Calculating the APGAR Score
Individual scores are summed to give a total ranging from 0 to 10, indicating the type of resuscitation needed. Make every effort to give an accurate score to the emergency room personnel.
- 7 to 10, no resuscitation needed;
- 4 to 6, stimulate, suction, and give oxygen;
- 0 to 3, begin ventilation and CPR.

Source: V.A. Apgar, "A Proposal for a New Method of Evaluation of the Newborn Infant," *Current Research in Anesthesia and Analgesia,* vol. 32 (1953), pp. 260–67.

Management

The prehospital provider should put on a gown, gloves, mask, and eye protection to reduce exposure to the mother's blood during the birth. BLS management of the newborn includes the following:

Airway Control

- As the head is delivered, inspect for the presence of the umbilical cord around the neck of the newborn and attempt to loosen and unwrap it if present. If it cannot be unwrapped, place two clamps on the cord and cut it between the clamps. Permitting the delivery to proceed without loosening the cord will asphyxiate the infant.
- After the head is delivered, suction the mouth two or three times **first,** and then the nose with a bulb syringe. Suctioning the nose first will often trigger spontaneous breathing and potential aspiration of the contents of the mouth. Remember to depress the bulb syringe before suctioning (Figure 14.1).
- Note the presence of green- or black-colored substance similar to thick pea soup, which is indicative of meconium. (See Caution box for management.)
- Hold the baby with the head in neutral position as delivery progresses, taking care not to drop the slippery infant.
- Wipe blood and mucus off the face and suction the mouth and nose again.

CAUTION!

MECONIUM STAINING AND ASPIRATION

When an infant's skin or the amniotic fluid has a dark greenish stain, the baby was distressed during labor or delivery. Meconium is a dark green-black, thick, sticky bowel movement. You may see the green-black staining as the baby's head emerges. Get prepared to suction the baby's mouth and nose while the head is being delivered. If meconium is in the mouth and airway and the infant breathes spontaneously prior to suctioning, aspiration of meconium will occur. These infants have a high mortality rate. The infant must be aggressively suctioned prior to stimulation of spontaneous breathing, even at the risk of causing bradycardia. BLS providers should use a mechanical suction device, such as a meconium aspirator, to remove thick meconium.

The ALS provider should examine the trachea with the laryngoscope and intubate the infant, followed by suctioning of the trachea if meconium is seen as soon as the infant is born. Artificial ventilation with 100% oxygen should be initiated as soon as most of the meconium is removed.

Temperature Control

- Dry the infant with a warmed towel. Discard the wet towel and wrap the baby in another warmed, dry towel or blanket. Cover the head. This stimulation frequently causes the baby to breathe spontaneously.

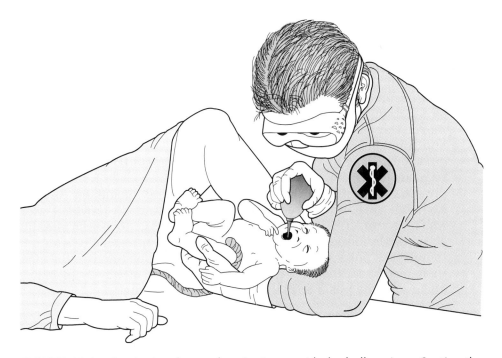

FIGURE 14.1   Suctioning the newborn's airway with the bulb syringe. Suction the mouth first and then the nose. Suctioning the nose first may trigger spontaneous breathing before the airway is clear of mucus or meconium.

- Place the infant on a warmed towel with the head lower than the trunk at the same level as the mother and cut the umbilical cord (Figure 14.2).
- If resuscitation is not necessary, have the mother hold the baby next to her bare skin.

FIGURE 14.2   After the infant has been dried, place in a clean, warmed towel with head slightly lower than the trunk prior to cutting the umbilical cord.

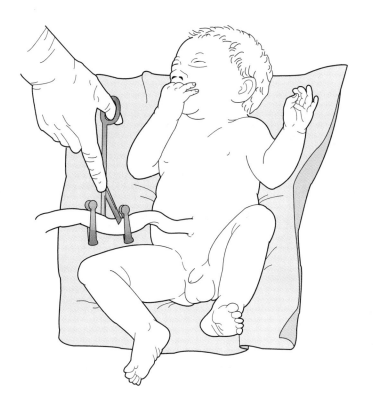

Care of the Newly Born Infant

Ventilations

- If breathing has not yet started, further stimulate the baby by flicking or slapping the feet and rubbing the back (Figure 14.3).
- Assess the breathing effort after 5–10 seconds.
- If no spontaneous breathing or gasping respirations occur after stimulation, artificial ventilation with a bag-valve mask must be initiated. Ventilate with high-flow, high-concentration oxygen (warmed and humidified if available) at a rate of 40–60 breaths/min. (See guidelines for use of oxygen on page 211.) The initial breath should be made with the pop-off valve of the bag-valve mask disabled. This provides enough pressure to open the lung tissue for oxygen exchange to occur. Subsequent breaths should be provided with less pressure, only enough to make the chest rise. Reassess after 30 seconds. Continue artificial ventilations if no improvement is found.
- Infants are obligate nose breathers; they do not breathe through their mouth unless they are crying or an oral airway is in place. Make sure the nasal passages remain clear of mucus.

Bradycardia

- Monitor the heart rate. Palpate the umbilical stump or the brachial pulse. If the heart rate is less than 100/min, continue bag-mask valve ventilation at a rate of 40–60/min with high-flow, high-concentration oxygen. The heart rate should increase within 15–30 seconds.
- If the heart rate is less than 60/min or between 60–80/min and not responding after 30 seconds of bag-mask ventilation, begin chest compressions. (See Chapter 5, "Pediatric Cardiopulmonary Resuscitation.")
- Rapidly transport the distressed infant to the hospital. A less urgent transport is needed for the stable mother and newborn. Position the baby on its side to prevent aspiration of secretions.
- Discontinue artificial ventilation but maintain blow-by oxygen when the infant breathes spontaneously and perfuses adequately and maintains a heart rate above 100/min.

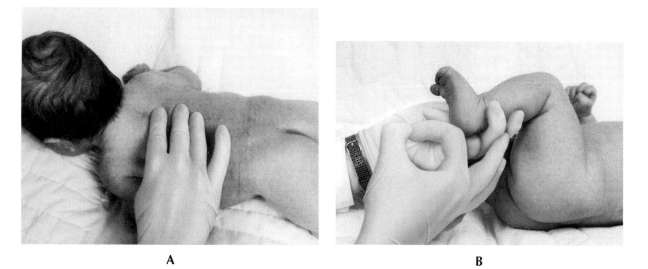

A **B**

FIGURE 14.3 *Stimulate breathing by (A) rubbing the infant's back or (B) flicking the feet.*

ALS providers should perform the following additional care to a distressed infant:

- Assess the approximate weight of the newborn.
- Intubate when there is no response to bag-mask ventilation and oxygen. Monitor the heart rate for further decreases in heart rate. Reoxygenate for 20 seconds with bag-mask ventilation if intubation takes longer than 30 seconds.
- Give epinephrine, 0.01–0.03 mg/kg/dose of 1:10,000 solution, by endotracheal tube or IV or IO if bradycardia does not respond to ventilation, oxygenation, and chest compressions.
- Depending upon local protocol, an IV can be started either with a peripheral line, umbilical cannulation, or intraosseous line. For hypovolemia, give 10 mL/kg of Ringer's Lactate or Normal Saline.
- Naloxone, 0.1 mg/kg IV, IO, or ET may be used in a nonresponsive newborn if the mother has recently taken or is suspected to have taken a narcotic.

Guidelines for the Use of Oxygen in Newborns

The newborn's brain cells are very sensitive to hypoxia, and permanent brain damage will result if hypoxemia is prolonged. For this reason, oxygen should never be withheld from a newborn suspected to have hypoxia.

Give oxygen by blow-by when bag-mask ventilation is not needed at 5–10 L/min flow rate. Use a bag-valve mask with reservoir when high-flow, high-concentration oxygen is needed for resuscitation.

Cold oxygen blown directly on the baby's face around the nose, in the distribution of the trigeminal nerve, will cause apnea. Apnea is triggered by the mammalian diving reflex. Warmed oxygen does not cause apnea. If cold blow-by oxygen is begin administered, direct the oxygen to the nose from one side of the baby's face (Figure 14.4). This will reduce the chances of triggering the diving reflex.

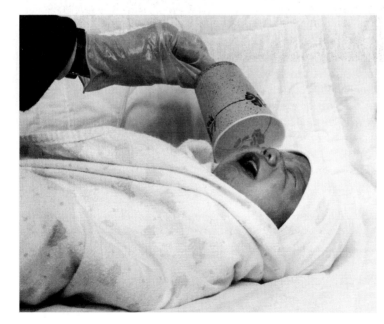

FIGURE 14.4   When oxygen cannot be warmed, direct the flow of oxygen to the nose from one side of the newborn's face rather than directly on the face around the nose. This will reduce the chance of triggering the mammalian diving reflex, which causes apnea.

Premature Infants

Premature infants are generally those born prior to 37 weeks of gestation. Their weight may range from 1.5 to 5 pounds (0.6–2.2 kg). Size of the newborn should not be the criteria used to begin resuscitation. Some fetuses are malnourished and very small, but they may be near full-term. It is also not possible to determine which small premature infants will survive. The lower limit of survival for premature infants is now 24–26 weeks when cared for in an intensive care nursery.

Assessment

The premature infant's degree of immaturity determines the physical characteristics seen on examination. The infant generally has a large trunk and shorter-appearing extremities, which maintain a frog-like position. The infant's skin is generally transparent and less wrinkled than is the skin of a full-term infant.

Management

- In the case of a very small infant, initiate resuscitation if the infant has any signs of life, such as breathing, movement, or a heart rate.
- Follow guidelines for management of the newborn on pages 208–211.
- Artificial ventilation is often required immediately after birth.
- Keep the infant well oxygenated and warm. Use insulated blankets, caps, or plastic wrap to help the infant retain body heat (Figure 14.5). Premature infants lose body heat more rapidly than full-term infants.
- Transport the infant to a hospital with specialized services for low birth-weight infants if available.

CAUTION!

OXYGEN USE IN LOW BIRTH-WEIGHT INFANTS

Low birth-weight infants are at risk for retrolental fibroplasia. Concentration of oxygen is one factor associated with the development of this disorder. However, the amount of oxygen used during routine prehospital transport is not believed to cause the condition. It is more important to ensure that the infant is *well oxygenated to prevent brain damage.* Administer enough oxygen to keep the infant pink and well perfused. Remember to keep the infant warm, which will also reduce oxygen demands.

ALS providers should have equipment that measures oxygen saturation levels for longer transport times. The concentration of oxygen to be administered to the low birth-weight infant can then be more precisely calculated.

Respiratory Distress in Newborns

Newborn respiratory distress is caused by a number of disorders, including the following:

- Obstruction of the nasal passages either by mucus or a congenital blockage (choanal atresia);

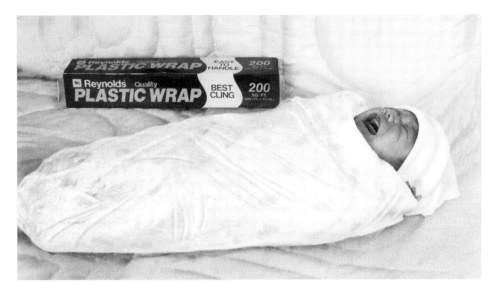

FIGURE 14.5   Keep small newborns warm during transport by wrapping them in insulated blankets or plastic wrap.

- Meconium aspiration;
- Amniotic fluid aspiration; and
- Lung immaturity.

Each of these problems could progress to cardiac arrest if appropriate intervention is not provided early for hypoxia.

Assessment

Signs of respiratory distress in the newborn include the following:

- See-saw or paradoxical breathing (the chest and abdomen do not rise and fall together with each breath; the chest rises as the abdomen falls and vice versa);
- Intercostal retractions;
- Nasal flaring; and
- Expiratory grunting that can be heard without a stethoscope.

Management

Prehospital care of the newborn in respiratory distress is the same as that provided to the normal newborn. Airway management and ventilation with high-flow, high-concentration oxygen must be well controlled. This infant needs immediate transport to the nearest hospital with the resources necessary for managing high-risk infants.

Newborn Management References

Banta, S.A., "Transition to extrauterine life," *Neonatal Network*, 3, (June 1985), pp. 35–39.

Chameides, L., and Hazinski, M.F., eds., *Textbook of Pediatric Advanced Life Support*, 2nd ed. Dallas: American Heart Association, 1994.

Dodman, N., "Newborn temperature control," *Neonatal Network*, 5, (June 1987), pp. 19–22.

Dunlap, T., "Grasping the principles of neonatal resuscitation," *JEMS*, 11, no. 1 (January 1994), pp. 46–57.

Emergency Cardiac Core Curriculum and Subcommittees, American Heart Association, "Guidelines for cardiopulmonary resuscitation and emergency care: VII Neonatal resuscitation," *JAMA*, 268, no. 16 (October 28, 1992), pp. 2276–2281.

Leuthner, S.R., Jansen, R.D., and Hageman, J.R., "Cardiopulmonary resuscitation of the newborn: An update," *Pediatric Clinics of North America*, 41, no. 5 (October 1994), pp. 893–907.

Silverman, B.J., ed., *Advanced Pediatric Life Support.* Dallas: American College of Emergency Physicians, 1994.

Apnea and Sudden Infant Death Syndrome

OBJECTIVES

When you have completed this chapter you should be able to

▶ Differentiate between sleep apnea and sudden infant death syndrome (SIDS).
▶ Describe the physical findings noted on the SIDS victim.
▶ List the current research findings associated with SIDS.
▶ Describe the parents' or caretakers reactions to the SIDS emergency.
▶ Describe the responsibilities of the EMS field providers in caring for the family experiencing a SIDS emergency.

Apnea and Apparent Life-Threatening Events

Apnea is a temporary prolonged pause in breathing, and when it is severe it places an infant at risk for recurrent hypoxia and hypoventilation. Newborns and infants commonly have short episodes of respiratory pause with spontaneous respiration interrupting the apnea. These episodes of *periodic breathing* lasts less than 20 seconds and are not considered to be abnormal.

Apnea of infancy is a condition in which the infant develops irregular and sporadic breathing patterns, generally lasting longer than 20 seconds. A shorter duration of apnea accompanied by signs of bradycardia, pallor, or cyanosis is also defined as apnea of infancy. These infants are believed to be at increased risk for sudden infant death syndrome (SIDS). Premature infants have a higher incidence of apnea, probably associated with immaturity of their respiratory and neurologic systems. Its occurrence is thought to peak between 1 month and 4 months of age.

Apnea is also defined by mechanism of breathing pause. In *central apnea* there is neither chest movement, muscle movement, nor air passing through the nose or mouth, because the infant is making no breathing effort. In cases of *obstructive apnea*, there is chest movement and the infant is trying to breathe, but an obstruction is blocking air movement. Often there is *mixed apnea*, a combination of the two types.

An *apparent life-threatening event* (ALTE) is an episode in infants, usually under 6 months of age, that is frightening to the observer. It is characterized by some combination of apnea (usually central but occasionally obstructive), color change, marked decrease in muscle tone, and choking or gagging. These episodes have previously been called "near miss SIDS." Research has identified only a small overlap between infants with ALTE who subsequently die of SIDS; however, there is an increased risk of SIDS among infants with ALTE. Those at greatest risk are infants requiring vigorous stimulation or resuscitation to terminate the episode of apnea.

ALTE is sometimes associated with neurologic problems, seizures, or gastroesophageal reflux; however, no cause of ALTE is found in half of the cases. It occurs in 0.5% to 0.6% of all infants, but approximately 7% of the premature infants.

History

Getting the patient history should not interfere with the resuscitation effort. Important information to obtain from the parent or care provider includes the following:

S Was the infant found limp and unresponsive or did someone observe a prolonged pause in breathing? Was the child's color blue? Did the infant cough or gag?

A Does the infant have any known allergies?

M Does the infant take any regular medications?

P Does the infant have any known medical problems or acute illness? Was the infant born prematurely? Has the infant had other episodes like this? When did the last one occur?

L When was the infant's last oral intake? What was it?

E Was the child stimulated or was resuscitation started prior to the arrival of EMS? What was the response to these efforts? Does the parent use an apnea monitor?

Assessment

During the initial assessment, the infant with an ALTE may appear lifeless with marked limpness, pallor or cyanosis, no respiratory effort, and no response to mild stimulation. Either bradycardia or no pulse will be detected. Alternately, the infant may have an irregular respiratory pattern with apnea spells longer than 20 seconds, choking, or gagging. The infant with some respirations will be pale, cyanotic or reddish, bradycardic, limp, but responsive to mild stimulation.

Management

BLS care for the infant with an ALTE includes the following:

- Assess and monitor ABCs.
- Administer high-flow, high-concentration oxygen and assist ventilations at 40 breaths/min.
- Initiate CPR if no heart rate is detected or if the infant's heart rate is less than 60 beats per minute after assisted ventilation and oxygen.
- Transport patient rapidly to nearest emergency department.
- If infant responds to stimulation or resuscitation with spontaneous regular respirations, continue high-flow, high-concentration oxygen while en route.
- Keep the infant warm.
- Provide reassurance to the parents that you are doing everything you can for the infant.

ALS providers may want to add the following management:

- Intubate immediately.
- Start an IV or IO line. Use Ringer's Lactate or Normal Saline at a keep-open rate.
- Attach a cardiac monitor and pulse oximeter.
- Initiate the PALS (Pediatric Advanced Life Support) drug protocol if the heart rate does not increase with oxygen or no pulse and/or no respiratory effort are present.

Sudden Infant Death Syndrome

Sudden infant death syndrome (SIDS), previously known as "crib death" or "cot death," is the sudden and unexplained death of an infant under one year of age. It is a distinct medical diagnosis made after the exclusion of all other causes of death after a thorough case investigation that includes a review of the clinical history, examination of the death scene, and a complete autopsy. The onset and death are believed to occur rapidly with no suffering and to be associated with sleep.

At the present time, SIDS is unpredictable and cannot be prevented. It is the leading cause of death of infants between 1 and 12 months of age; 4,891 infants died from SIDS in the United States in 1992. However, progress has been made. Between 1993 and 1995, it is estimated that the number of deaths due to SIDS decreased 30%. This has been linked to the new recommendation that infants be put to sleep on their back, rather than on their side or stomach.

Research has revealed common characteristics of SIDS infants and its occurrence. SIDS occurs more often in the fall and winter months. The peak age for SIDS is between 2 and 4 months, and the majority of cases occur before 7 months of age. Death usually occurs during sleep. Infants believed to be at higher risk for SIDS include the following:

- Male (60% of cases);
- Infants exposed to second-hand smoke;
- Infants sleeping on stomach;
- Infants wearing excess clothing;
- Low birth-weight infants (4 times more frequent);
- Infants of young unmarried mothers of low socioeconomic status, even though it occurs in families of all socioeconomic levels;
- Infants of mothers who did not receive adequate prenatal care; who smoked cigarettes or used cocaine, methadone, or heroin during pregnancy; and who have a history of sexually transmitted disease or urinary tract infection.

Reducing Risk Factors Associated with SIDS

- Place healthy babies on their back to sleep, especially during the first 6 months of life. This practice has resulted in an estimated 30% reduction in the rate of SIDS death between 1993 and 1995.
- Do not smoke around babies because constant exposure to smoke doubles or triples the baby's risk of SIDS.
- Use firm bedding materials. Avoid sheepskins, foam pads or cushions, pillows, and waterbeds.
- Avoid overheating babies with too much clothing or too much bedding. Keep babies dressed with the same amount of clothing worn by others in the home.
- Breast-feed babies, if possible, which helps prevent gastrointestinal and respiratory illnesses and other infections.

History

Questions should be phrased so blame is not implied. Questions should not include "you," such as "When did you. . . ?" The parents will already feel guilty, and such questions will make them take on additional blame. If open-ended questions are used, such as "What happened?" most of the necessary information will be provided.

- Who discovered the infant; when and where?
- What action was taken by that person?
- When was the baby put to bed, or when did the baby fall asleep?
- What is the age and weight of the infant?
- What has the baby's general health been like? Have there been any recent illnesses? When was the child last seen by the doctor?
- Were there any health problems identified in the baby at birth?

Assessment

EMS will be activated when the parent or care provider finds the infant lifeless with no pulse or respiratory effort. The baby will be cool or cold if adequate time has elapsed since death. The infant may be limp, or stiff if rigor mortis is present. Lividity or purple marks may be noted on the dependent parts of the body where blood has settled.

By the time the EMTs arrive, the parents may have picked up the infant and/or initiated CPR. If the infant is still lying in the crib, the following signs are usually present:

Chapter 15: Apnea and Sudden Infant Death Syndrome

- No evidence of having been disturbed during sleep, or the infant may have changed position at the time of death. It is not uncommon for infants to be found wedged in the corner of the crib.
- Blood-tinged fluid around the mouth and nose or on bed covers. This discharge is associated with muscle relaxation after death rather than vomitus, which could have caused an airway obstruction.
- The infant's head may be covered with a blanket; however, suffocation has been ruled out as a cause of death in these infants because oxygen levels were adequate to sustain life.

Parents may demonstrate a wide range of behavior to emergency personnel. Most are anxious for help in saving their infant. When the parent suspects the infant is dead or has it confirmed, a number of grief reactions are possible, including the following:

- Shock, disbelief, denial (they do not recognize the reality of the situation);
- Hysteria;
- Inability to make decisions; disorganization and difficulty functioning;
- Guilt and self-blame;
- Withdrawal and depression.

Management

Emergency care in the case of an apparently dead infant, assumed to be the victim of SIDS, is to be supportive of the parents and assist them in the grieving process. Often BLS and ALS providers will follow the same protocols, especially when death occurred hours earlier. Parents will be helped the most if they feel that everything possible was done to save their infant.

- Assess and monitor ABCs.
- Initiate CPR, usually with BLS maneuvers according to medical direction. (This action is not taken in some jurisdictions when signs indicate death occurred hours earlier.)
- Even when you have limited or no hope of successful resuscitation, support the parents and demonstrate your concern by explaining what is being done. Do not offer false hope that the infant will recover. Parents will have selective memory of the entire resuscitation episode. Your gestures to help the child and offer the parents some assistance will be remembered, even if the details are forgotten.
- Transport the infant and parent(s) to the hospital if local guidelines permit. If the parent cannot be transported in the ambulance, arrange for other transport. Parents are too distraught to drive themselves.
- If possible when at the hospital, try to offer some comfort to the parents by sitting with them; while the infant is cared for by hospital personnel, listen to the parents if they want to talk, offer to make phone calls for them, etc.
- If local protocol does not permit transport of the dead infant to the hospital, such as when the coroner is called to the scene, do not leave the parents alone in the home with the dead infant. If the rescue squad must leave, arrange for a neighbor, family member, or the clergy to stay with the parents until the coroner arrives.

In the recent past, infants initially thought to be victims of child abuse have later been determined to be SIDS victims. Parents were subjected to accusations and criminal investigations, which obstructed their grieving process. Overdiagnosis of SIDS in infants who could possibly be victims of child abuse is still a controversial subject. Concrete evidence from the autopsy and the scene to diagnose child abuse has not been present in these cases, but circumstantial evidence has made many people suspect it. (See Table 15.1 to distinguish between signs of SIDS and child abuse.) Child abuse is another major cause of death in infants, and it is important to be alert to the possibility. However, do not make judgments about the infant's cause of death or indirectly blame the parents for the child's death.

Assessment

Make a thorough assessment of the scene, noting any discrepancies among the history, the environment, the behavior of the parents, and your assessment of the infant. Observations to make when you are suspicious of child abuse include the following:

- Physical appearance of the baby, especially before CPR is initiated. If the parents initiated first aid, this may account for some of the marks on the body.
- The position of the baby in the crib may account for marks noted on the child's head and body, such as lividity in dependent body parts or pressure marks from lying against side rails.
- Physical appearance of the crib and objects in the crib.
- Unusual or dangerous items in the room (sharp objects, plastic bags).
- Behaviors of people present.
- Medications or drugs that are present; intended for the infant or adult. (You may choose to take medications to the hospital.)
- Appearance of the room and house.

Management

Regardless of your suspicions of child abuse, the resuscitation effort must begin. All prehospital providers should perform the following care:

- *DO NOT* delay treatment or transport to make the scene investigation.
- Report your findings objectively, not your assumptions about the case, based upon evidence seen. All information should be objectively and factually documented in the official prehospital report. Your suspicions and objective information should be reported confidentially to the emergency department staff at the receiving hospital.
- Notify local authorities. Let the police do the investigation; your job is to care for the family.

Apnea and SIDS References

Barkin, R.M., and Rosen, P., eds., *Emergency Pediatrics*, 4th ed. St. Louis: Mosby Year Book, Inc., 1994.

Bass, M., Kravath, R.E., and Glass, L., "Death scene investigation in sudden infant death," *New England Journal of Medicine*, 315, no. 2 (1986), pp. 100–105.

TABLE 15.1 ■ *Distinguishing Characteristics of SIDS and Child Abuse/Neglect*

SUDDEN INFANT DEATH SYNDROME	CHILD ABUSE AND NEGLECT
Incidence: Deaths: 6500–7500/year Highest: 2 to 4 months of age When: Winter months	*Incidence:* Deaths: 1000–4000/year Deaths in infants: 300/year When: No seasonal difference
Physical Appearance: Exhibits no external signs of injury Exhibits "natural" appearance of dead baby: • Lividity—settling of blood; frothy draining from nose/mouth • Small marks, e.g., diaper rash looks more severe • Cooling/rigor mortis—takes place quickly in infants (about 3 hours) Appears to be well-developed baby, though may be small for age	*Physical Appearance:* Distinguishable and visible signs of injury • Broken bone(s) • Bruises • Burns • Cuts • Head trauma (black eye) • Scars • Welts • Wounds May have no external signs of injury May be obviously malnourished Other siblings may show patterns of injuries commonly seen in child abuse

May Initially Suspect SIDS:
All of the above characteristics
    PLUS
Parents say that infant was well and healthy when put to sleep (last time seen alive).
	May Initially Suspect Child Abuse or Neglect:
	All of the above characteristics
	    PLUS
	Parents' story does not "sound right" or cannot account for all of injuries on infant.

Source: Adapted from Bureau of Community Health Services (HSA/PHS). *Training Emergency Responders: Sudden Infant Death Syndrome, An Instructor's Manual.* 1979. p. C–3. Used with permission, National SIDS Clearinghouse.

Brooks, J.G., "Apparent life-threatening events and apnea of infancy," *Clinics in Perinatology,* 19, no. 4 (December 1992), pp. 809–838.

Carlson, J.A., "The psychologic effects of Sudden Infant Death Syndrome on parents," *Journal of Pediatric Health Care,* 7, no. 2 (March/April 1993), pp. 77–81.

Havens, D.H., and Zink, R.L., "The `Back to Sleep' campaign," *Journal of Pediatric Health Care,* 8, no. 5 (September/October 1994), pp. 240–242.

Hellmich, H., "Sleeping on back helps cut SIDS deaths 30%," *USA Today* (June 25, 1996), p. A1.

Herda, J.A., "Nursing interventions aimed at reducing the risks of SIDS," *Pediatric Nursing,* 18, no. 5 (September/October 1992), pp. 531–533.

Lawrence, D., "SIDS: Handle with care," *JEMS,* 13, no. 12 (December 1988), pp. 51–53.

Morbidity and Mortality Weekly Report, "Infant mortality—United States, 1992," *Morbidity and Mortality Weekly Report,* 43, no. 49 (December 16, 1994), pp. 905–909.

Sudden Infant Death Syndrome: Trying to Understand the Mystery. McLean, VA: National Sudden Infant Death Resource Center, USDHHS, PHS, HRSA, MCHB, 1994.

Suicide in Children and Adolescents

OBJECTIVES

When you have completed this chapter you should be able to

▶ Recognize the potential of a suicide attempt or gesture in the child or adolescent.
▶ Describe appropriate ways to communicate with the suicidal child or adolescent.

Suicide and Suicide Attempts

Suicide and *suicide attempts* are difficult situations to handle when the patient is an adult. However, it becomes an incomprehensible and highly charged emotional event when the person is a child or an adolescent. You must be able to recognize potential suicidal behavior in the child. Recognition, evaluation, and documentation of this behavior are vital to receiving hospital personnel. Rapid decisions and referrals for psychosocial intervention must be made early to assure the child's protection from further harmful acts.

Suicide is a self-inflicted injury that results in death. A *suicide attempt* or *gesture* refers to an attention-seeking behavior that threatens suicide often without any real effort to die. All suicide attempts or gestures must be taken seriously, and the child should be considered at high risk for further suicidal behavior.

Epidemiology

Incidence

- Suicide has been identified in preschoolers as young as 2½ years of age.
- In 1991, 1899 adolescents between 10 to 14 years of age and 2852 adolescents between 15 and 19 years of age took their own lives.
- The suicide rate increases for youth as they progress to adulthood. For youths between 15 and 19 years of age, the suicide rate has tripled over the last three decades, and it is now the third leading cause of death for this age group.
- Males commit suicide four times more frequently than females in all age groups. However, more males than females 12 years of age and under will attempt suicide; the sex distribution reverses itself after 12 years of age.
- The suicide rate is equally distributed among all socioeconomic groups. It is more common in white teens than nonwhite teens. The risk is higher for teens who are unemployed or married.
- In 1993, 24% of U.S. high-school students seriously considered attempting suicide, and more than 8% actually made the attempt.

The actual number of suicides in children is unknown for a variety of reasons. Many suicides are masked as "accidents," such as single-car crashes with the driver as the only passenger. Ingestions of poisons in children 5 years of age and older are highly suspicious. Parents may actually try to conceal suicide attempts because of strong feelings of failure and guilt, denial, and a tendency to minimize the suicidal ideations of their children.

Physicians and medical examiners are often unwilling to record suicide as a cause of death owing to a lack of clear-cut evidence or to keep from stigmatizing the parents. Sometimes the parents themselves will request that suicide not be recorded on the death certificate.

Mechanism of Injury

The methods that children will use to commit or attempt suicide vary by age group. Children 10 years of age or under will, typically, stab themselves or set themselves on fire. Older children and adolescents commonly use firearms (especially males), hanging, self-poisoning, and single-car crashes as the method. According to a recent study, 70% of adolescents who are successful or failed suicide victims chose firearms as the method. Further evidence shows that suicide by firearms is directly related to their availability.

Psychosocial Risk Factors

Factors that precipitate suicidal behavior or a suicide attempt include some type of interpersonal conflict or interpersonal loss. Disruptions within the family often contribute to suicide ideations in the younger child. Disruptions outside the family unit often increase in significance as the child gets older (Table 16.1).

Risk factors for suicide include depression, shame, and feelings of being unable to live up to expectations. Shame could be associated with physical or sexual abuse or legal or disciplinary problems. Teens may be depressed and believe there are only two options—to be miserable for the rest of their lives, or to die.

Adolescents attempting suicide may be exhibiting manipulative behavior. Their purpose may include any of the following:

- to inflict revenge on someone,
- to increase their power or to manipulate others to their favor,
- to gain attention, or
- to escape a difficult situation.

Developmental Concepts of Death and Related Suicidal Ideations

Under 3 Years of Age

Infants and toddlers, up to about 3 years of age, view death as separation.

3 to 7 Years of Age

Children from 3 to 7 years of age are unable to grasp death as permanent and will personify death; for example, death is a wicked witch or a monster in the closet. During a crisis, death may be viewed as desirable and a temporary means of escape. Children may even fantasize about their

TABLE 16.1 ■ *Psychosocial Risk Factors of Suicide Behavior in Children and Adolescents*

FAMILY INFLUENCES	OTHER SOCIETAL INFLUENCES
Divorce	Loss of love relationship
Death of parent or other family member (sibling, grandparent)	Peer pressure
	Fear of being different
Separation—actual or threatened	Low self-esteem
Rejection—real or imagined	Graduation from high school
Child abuse or neglect	Drug abuse
	Uncertainty about future
	Imitation-contagion theory
	Depression
	Legal Problems

own death. For example, they fantasize themselves lying in a coffin while family members are crying and wishing them back to life, making statements such as, "I should never have yelled at her, and if she comes back I'll give her everything she wants." This age group is incapable, developmentally, of skills of strategy and foresight. This is particularly dangerous because it leads to impulsive behavior.

7 to 12 Years of Age

Children initially begin to grasp the permanency of death between 7 and 12 years of age; however, 50% of 12-year-olds still believe death is not permanent, but reversible. This age group does not differentiate between thoughts and actions; therefore, they view suicidal thoughts and actions as the same thing. They are developmentally capable of strategy and foresight and will premeditate, or plan, when and how to commit suicide.

12 Years Through Adolescence

Adolescents generally begin to recognize that death is permanent. It is important to remember that this age group is exposed to high family stress as well as increasing peer group and societal stress, which puts them at higher risk for suicide than any other age group.

CAUTION!

> Children may vary from the development ages listed above owing to a variety of environmental factors and life experiences. The sex of the child can also determine his/her emotional and developmental level at any particular age. Therefore, the individual child should be considered when doing your assessment, using the above information only as a guide.

Common Misconceptions About Suicide

There are many misconceptions about suicide that apply to all age groups. Becoming aware of these is key to the complete management of the suicidal child. Some of the most common misconceptions are listed below.

Those Who Talk About Suicide Never Do It

Many children will make an attempt, usually verbally, to let someone know. They may not come right out and say "I'm going to kill myself"; rather, they may say, "I want to die" or "Nobody cares about me anyway." *Take these statements seriously! They are a cry for help!*

Suicide Happens Without Warning

Numerous hints or warnings are often given either verbally or in the form of gestures, such as becoming accident prone or taking only a few pills. The child may give away cherished belongings to a friend or sibling. These are nonverbal clues to suicide ideations.

Once Suicidal, Always Suicidal

There is a 24–72 hour peak danger period following a suicide risk crisis. Children tend to believe that the pain they are feeling will continue forever.

They do not have the life experiences to recall and remember that the pain they are feeling is temporary and will eventually subside, probably within a few days.

Once an Attempt Is Survived, There Will Never Be Another Attempt

There is a high risk for future attempts if prior attempts are not followed by psychological intervention. Future attempts become more lethal and usually occur within a year of the first attempt. You can reduce the chance of future attempts by relaying pertinent information to the appropriate medical personnel so that psychosocial intervention can begin early in the child's medical care.

Suicide Victims Always Leave Notes

Only a small number of individuals leave notes. This is one of the reasons why many suicides are classified as accidents.

Never Use the Word "Suicide" When Talking with Children: It May Give Them the Idea

The word *suicide* won't put the idea into the mind of a child who is not suicidal. Using the word can actually invite the suicidal child to verbalize feelings of despair. It can help establish rapport and trust by showing the child that you are taking his or her feelings seriously.

Suicide Is Hereditary

Though the tendency may be increased in a family with a prior suicide, it is not genetically inherited. A child may view the suicide of a family member as an appropriate way to solve a problem. Typically, children have not yet learned how to cope effectively, reduce stress, and work toward a more promising future.

History

A complete history should be obtained from the child and any available family members. Listen and communicate directly with the child, whenever possible. Talking with the child may promote building trust and rapport with the child. Some questions to use that will help you identify the child with suicidal thoughts include: (Brent, 1989)

- Have you ever thought that life was not worth living?
- Have you ever wished you were dead?
- Have you ever thought about trying to hurt yourself?
- Do you intend to hurt yourself? How? (This might alert the EMS provider to the presence of a weapon.)
- Do you have a plan to hurt yourself?
- Have you ever attempted suicide?

If a family member hinders your efforts to obtain information about suicidal behaviors, you may have to separate the child from this person. Do this in a calm and compassionate manner. Transport the child as soon as the opportunity presents itself. The family member can ride in the front of the ambulance while you talk with the child en route to the emergency department.

Assessment

Note and document all pertinent information heard and observed at the scene. Was a mechanism of injury present, such as pill bottles, a firearm, or rope? Was a note left? If a danger exists, then scene safety is a priority. Consider police involvement.

Some additional information that can be collected and used *to evaluate the child's severity of suicidal risk* at this time, such as the High Risk-Low Rescue Factors, are listed below. An answer of "yes" to any or all of the questions shows that the child is at high risk. The child did not intend to be rescued.

High Risk-Low Rescue Factors

- Did the attempt take place in isolation and at a time when discovery was unlikely?
- Did the child not seek help before, during, or after the attempt?
- Was a final act performed; for example, did the child give away cherished possessions?
- Was the expected outcome death, i.e., choice of an irreversible method?
- Did the child plan ahead to commit suicide?
- Was a suicide note written?

Management

ALS and BLS providers must provide prompt care when treating the self-inflicted injury as well as offer psychological support during transport.

- Size-up the scene.
- Assess and monitor ABCs.
- Manage all life-threatening injuries.
- Use caution to preserve evidence for potential police investigation. You may need to request police backup.
- Transport the child with parents whenever possible.
- Remember to document and pass on both medical reports and discussions with the child to the receiving hospital personnel.

Psychological Support During Management and Transport

Provide psychological support to the child, using the following guidelines of appropriate interventions.

- Ensure a safe environment.
- Isolate the child from tension and provocation. Move the child to a private area whenever possible.
- Take the child's threats seriously. This will help gain the child's trust and assist you in establishing rapport with the child. It is possible that you may be the first person that has paid attention to the patient's feelings.
- Listen with interest and sensitivity. Only one responder should work directly with the child. Others should remain present but silent.
- Offer support, understanding, and compassion for what the child is telling you. Let the child know that you are there to help.
- Acknowledge the child's feelings. This does not mean that you agree with the child's actions but you can relate, to some degree, to the child's feelings of hopelessness and despair. Avoid making statements such as "I know how you feel" as this may bring out a nega-

tive response. Instead, say something to the effect of, "I understand why you feel so lonely" or "That must have made you very sad."

- Question the child about the attempt. Ask what happened to make life so difficult, and where the pills, gun, etc., come from. Ask children who attempt suicide why they did what they did and what they thought would happen. Find out when they first thought about doing this and if they ever attempted suicide in the past. If they tell you they have attempted suicide in the past, find out when. Find out if there is anyone to stop them. They may be alone most of the time.

Avoid the following inappropriate behaviors or actions when caring for the suicidal child.

- *DO NOT* act judgmental, either verbally or nonverbally. Examples of this are saying something to the effect of: "Why would you do such a silly thing?" or "You're such a pretty girl, and you have so much to live for." Rolling your eyes at a response is an example of non-verbal judgmental behavior.
- *DO NOT* make moral judgments. While the situation that caused the child's suicidal behavior may seem silly to you, it is very real and painful to the child. Children cannot rationalize situations like adults can because they lack experience in coping with difficult situations.
- *DO NOT* make light of the situation.
- *DO NOT* argue with the child about his or her feelings. Examples of this are saying something to the effect that "You don't really feel that way." Obviously the child does or he or she would not attempt to commit suicide.
- *DO NOT* discount the child's desire to die. For example, you can say "It's OK to feel like you want to die, but to try to kill yourself is not acceptable." This is the difference between feelings and actions, which is a difficult concept for children to understand.

Reactions of the EMS Provider

It is common for the prehospital care provider to have a very strong emotional reaction associated with a suicide or attempted suicide, especially when it involves a child. You may feel anger, both toward the child and the parents, as well as depression or anxiety. Helplessness is a common emotion EMTs and other people feel when someone contemplates suicide or actually commits the act.

Finally, it is of utmost importance to your emotional well-being to remember that it is not within your power to keep someone from committing suicide if that person really wants to die. Do not accept responsibility for someone's actions beyond providing that individual with the best medical care you are able to provide. (Consult Chapter 17, "Crisis and Stress Management," for assistance with your response to this type of rescue.)

Suicide References

Brent, D.A., "Depression and suicide in children and adolescents," *Pediatrics in Review*, 14 (October 1993), pp. 380–388.

_____ . "Suicide and suicide behavior in children and adolescents," *Pediatrics in Review*, 10 (1989), pp. 269–276.

Capuzzi, D., "Adolescent suicide: Prevention and intervention," *Counseling and Human Development*, 19, no. 2 (1986), pp. 1–9.

National Adolescent Health Information Center, *Fact sheet on adolescent suicide,* San Francisco: University of California, 1995.

Rickert, V.I., Porter-Levy, S., Levy, R.I., and Rickert, C.P., "Psychological and psychiatric emergencies: Strategies for providers," *Adolescent Medicine: State of the Art Reviews,* 4, no. 1 (February 1993), pp. 193–202.

Valente, S.M., "Assessing suicide risk in the school-age child," *Journal of Pediatric Health Care,* 1, no. 1 (January/February 1987), pp. 14–20.

Weisman, A.D., et al., "Risk-rescue rating in suicide assessment," *Archives of General Psychiatry,* 26, (June 1972), pp. 553–560.

Crisis and Stress Management

OBJECTIVES

When you have completed this chapter you should be able to

- ▶ Identify the psychological hazards of the EMS profession.
- ▶ Describe the differences among acute, delayed, and cumulative stress reactions.
- ▶ Describe the coping strategies that help reduce stress before, during, and after an event.

EMS providers by nature are very committed to their jobs and the patients they care for. They dedicate enormous numbers of hours, in addition to their regular jobs, as professional volunteers. Often, paid EMS professionals volunteer after hours on a unit in their community. These are people who place themselves at risk for a high level of stress in their lives. This stress should not automatically be considered harmful stress, unless the providers do not recognize and accept its existence or that their reactions to it are normal. Learned coping mechanisms and techniques for stress management make the difference between surviving stress or being harmed by it.

Characteristics of the EMS Profession

Personalities

EMS professionals are action oriented, like to be needed, and have a high level of energy. They are willing to take risks, make sacrifices, and do not give up easily, even when faced with overwhelming odds. They like to maintain control and are sensitive, yet many have learned to suppress their emotions to events that those outside of the profession cannot.

Job Qualities

Many aspects of the EMS profession can be considered exhilarating. It is a profession that attracts specially trained personnel and tests them beyond the breaking point, causing them to feel elite when they are successful. However, these are the very qualities that can create high levels of stress and stressful environments. For example, consider the following scenario: The scene is such that your abilities are tested to their limit; the child is seriously injured, and the management of the scene is difficult. There is a long extrication, and bystanders are hard to handle, *yet the child survives.* You can be left feeling elite and good about yourself, your coworkers, and the work you do. You feel great personal reward for your efforts.

But how often does the scenario described above occur? How often were you told, early on in your career, that a "save" is the exception rather than the rule? More often than not the scenario goes more like this: The scene is a difficult one, with bystanders pulling and yelling at you. The weather is miserable; it's cold or hot, it's pouring rain or snowing. Then the rescue takes longer than usual. The last crew shift did not have time to restock the ambulance, and you are missing necessary supplies. You need and use every skill you've ever learned, but the child is going downhill fast. You've been pushed to the limit of your endurance and you've met the challenge, but the child doesn't survive.

Both scenarios create stress; the difference is that the first resulted in a positive response to that stress; the second created a negative response, leaving you feeling angry, frustrated, and unsure of yourself and your abilities.

Occupational Hazards

As was mentioned in the chapters on child abuse and suicide, dealing with children can intensify your stress reactions, especially if the event results in death or injury from abuse, neglect, or suicide. However, children in general rank high on the list of occupational hazards for EMS providers that create a high degree of stress attributable to a variety of emotional and societal factors.

Children bring out the protective side of adults, whether they are parents or not. Children are cute, small, and vulnerable, evoking our sense of responsibility and desire to take care of them. They are young and we envision them growing up, not dying. Our society places a higher value on children; they are our future. Our feelings tend to come closer to the surface when confronted with a child, and these feelings are intensified when a child's life is at risk. Many EMS professionals have reported that becoming a parent themselves increased their level of stress reaction to ill and injured children. These are some of the underlying emotional and societal factors that create an environment that sets us up for stronger-than-normal stress reactions. Additionally, the injury or death of someone you know, the injury or death of one of your own colleagues, or any event that draws extraordinary media coverage also ranks high on the list of events that can create high stress.

> Stress must be recognized as a real potential for disrupting your mental health and well-being. It must be accepted as a real part of EMS, and when combined with stressful events related to family, friends, and/or additional jobs, the reaction to the stress of a particular event, or chain of events, increases.

CAUTION!

Types of Stress

Acute Stress

Acute stress is triggered by a critical event that happens during the rescue effort. It can cause a complete or partial mental or emotional breakdown. In very extreme cases, it may result in cardiac arrest. Symptoms can include physical, cognitive, and emotional reactions. See Table 17.1 for the range of signs and symptoms commonly identified. Not everyone will respond to the same incident in the same way. Stress is a normal reaction to an abnormal situation.

TABLE 17.1 ■ *Signs and Symptoms of Acute Stress Reaction*

PHYSICAL	COGNITIVE	EMOTIONAL
Nausea and upset stomach	Impaired thinking and decision making	Anxiety
Profuse sweating and tremors	Poor concentration and confusion	Fear
Dizziness and disorientation	Difficulty performing calculations	Grief and depression
Lack of coordination	Loss of memory	Feeling lost and abandoned
Increased heart rate	Concentration problems	Withdrawal
Increased blood pressure	Flashbacks	Anger
Headaches, muscle soreness	Poor attention span	Feeling shocked, numb,
Difficulty sleeping		and overwhelmed

Source: Mitchell, J.T., and Everly, G.S. (1994): *Signs and Symptoms of Acute Stress.* International Critical Incident Stress Foundation.

Delayed Posttraumatic Stress

Delayed stress reactions can occur minutes to weeks, months, or sometimes years after a stressful event. Signs and symptoms of a delayed stress reaction include the following:

- Increased feelings of anxiety, depression, and irritability;
- Sleep disturbances;
- Changes in eating habits;
- Loss of emotional control;
- Thoughts of suicide;
- Feelings of isolation;
- Decreased sexual drive and menstrual cycle changes;
- Decreased interest in family, significant others, friends;
- Increased marital disharmony;
- Changes in personality and behavior;
- Flashbacks;
- Marked differences in job performance.

There are three primary characteristics of delayed posttraumatic stress:

- Intrusive mental images. These can be in the form of dreams, nightmares, or flashbacks.
- Fear of repetition of the event, either real or imagined. The event remains so powerful that one begins to avoid activities associated with the event.
- Physical and emotional symptoms include sleep disturbances, fatigue, depression, and irritability.

Cumulative Stress

Cumulative stress is a state of chronic fatigue and frustration resulting from many disappointments and unrelieved stress. It is sometimes referred to as "burnout" and is difficult to differentiate from clinical depression. Signs and symptoms of cumulative stress include the following:

- Depression;
- Fatigue;
- Irritability;
- Apathy and disillusionment;
- Excessive defensiveness and withdrawal;
- Increased use of alcohol and drug abuse;
- Loss of energy;
- Increased illness.

Management and Coping Skills

The following guidelines can help you manage and cope with the stress associated with the emotionally charged work you perform daily.

- Obtain extensive EMS training; being current and well prepared can help prevent additional stress.
- Be part of a team; it can help reduce feelings of isolation (Figure 17.1).
- Improve communication skills and stress-management techniques.
- Utilize social and psychological support groups.
- Learn deep-breathing skills; this helps to diffuse tension and increase attention.

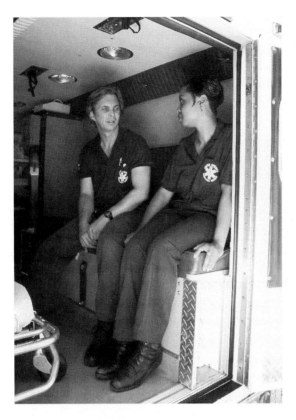

FIGURE 17.1 *When a particularly stressful call has been completed, make sure you talk about it with a trusted partner. Talking about your feelings will help reduce the impact of the stressful experience.*

- Use physical exercise, brisk walking, jogging, or calisthenics as a method to reduce a stress reaction. This should be done within a few hours after an event.
- East healthy meals, high in vitamins and protein.
- Try to maintain a normal schedule and avoid boredom.
- Express your feelings appropriately.
- Attend a Critical Incident Stress Debriefing when warranted.

The following actions may interfere with your ability to cope with stress.

- *DO NOT* use excessive humor to break tension. It may be misunderstood by bystanders and colleagues.
- *DO NOT* exaggerate efforts to control your emotions. Expressing emotions is healthier than suppressing them.
- *DO NOT* consume alcohol and/or drugs or use tobacco; they will only temporarily mask a stress response.
- *DO NOT* consume large doses of nicotine, caffeine, or sugar; they can heighten your stress reaction.
- *DO NOT* fight too hard against dreams and flashbacks; they are a normal response to a stressful event and will diminish over time.

Critical Incident Stress Debriefings (CISDs)

CISDs are a psychological and educational group process designed to reduce the impact of major events on EMS personnel and to accelerate normal recovery in normal people who are experiencing normal stress after experiencing highly abnormal events. A CISD is a reactive process since it is scheduled only after a stress-producing event occurs. Initiation of a CISD is dependent upon those who actually need the services requesting the meeting, unless the event was very significant.

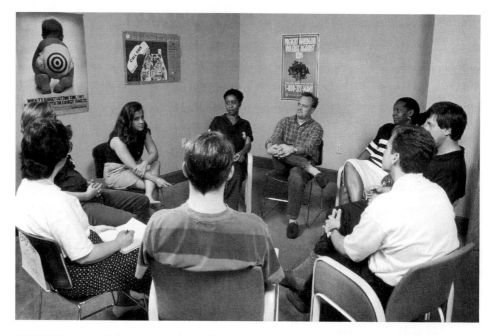

FIGURE 17.2   Take part in Critical Incidence Stress Debriefings when offered. Sharing feelings that several providers experienced will help confirm that your responses were normal to the abnormal situation.

CISDs are group sessions for everyone involved in the stressful event. They are conducted by one or two mental health professionals and peer-support personnel who have been trained to assist the group to express their feelings and work through stressful events in EMS (Figure 17.2). CISDs are held within 24 to 72 hours after the event, and attendance is voluntary.

If a Critical Incident Stress Debriefing is not offered after a highly stressful event, request one. If you are experiencing signs and symptoms of stress, it is likely that others involved in the incident are also experiencing them. If your symptoms persist beyond 6 weeks, seek additional help from a mental health professional experienced in crisis intervention and/or EMS providers and the problems they encounter in the field. Remember, without appropriate intervention a stress reaction can become damaging to your mental health and well-being.

Crisis and Stress References

Asken, M.J., *Psyche Response: Psychological Skills for Optimal Performance by Emergency Responders.* Englewood Cliffs, NJ: Prentice Hall, 1993.

Bassuk, E.L., et al., *Behavioral Emergencies: A Field Guide for EMTs and Paramedics.* Boston: Little Brown, 1983.

Boudreaux, E., Mandry, C., and Brantley, P.J., "Awake and hassled: What stresses an EMT," *JEMS,* 20 (November 1995), pp. 50–52.

Mitchell, J.T., and Bray, G.P., *Emergency Service Stress: Guidelines for Preserving the Health and Careers of Emergency Services Personnel.* Englewood Cliffs, NJ: Prentice Hall, 1990.

Mitchell, J.T., "Medic suicide: What can be done?" *JEMS,* 20 (November 1995) pp. 41–43.

Thomas, J.L., and Towberman, D.B., "Responding to the child within: Child abuse and the EMS provider," *JEMS,* 17 (March 1992), pp. 98–108.

Index